The SURRENDER

Also by Toni Bentley

Winter Season: A Dancer's Journal

Holding On to the Air: An Autobiography
(by Suzanne Farrell with Toni Bentley)

Costumes by Karinska

Sisters of Salome

The

SURRENDER

An Erotic Memoir

Toni Bentley

10 ReganBooks
Celebrating Ten Bestselling Years
An Imprint of HarperCollins*Publishers*

HarperCollins books may be purchased for educational, business, or sales promotional use. For information please write: Special Markets Department, HarperCollins Publishers Inc., 10 East 53rd Street, New York, NY 10022.

FIRST EDITION

Designed by Kris Tobiassen
Cover painting by John Kacere

Printed on acid-free paper

Library of Congress Cataloging-in-Publication Data
  Bentley, Toni.
      The surrender : an erotic memoir / Toni Bentley.—1st ed.
        p.   cm.
      ISBN 0-06-073246-6
      1. Bentley, Toni. 2. Women—United States—Sexual behavior—
Case studies. 3. Women—United States—Biography. 4. Ballet
dancers—United States—Biography. 5. Anal sex. I. Title.
HQ29.B45 2004
306.77—dc22
  [B]   2004050807

04 05 06 07 08 RRD 10 9 8 7 6 5 4 3

Virginia Woolf believed that no woman had succeeded in writing the truth of the experience of her own body—that women and language both would have to change considerably before anything like that could happen.

—CLAUDIA ROTH PIERPONT

I once loved a man so much that I no longer existed—all Him, no Me. Now I love myself just enough that no man exists—all Me, no Them. They all used to be God, and I used to be a figment of my own imagination; now men are figments of my imagination. Same game, different positions. I don't know how to play any other way. Someone must be on top, someone on bottom. Side by side is a bore. I tried it once for a few wildly disorienting minutes. Equality negates progress, prevents action. But a top and a bottom, well, they can get to the moon and back before equals can negotiate who pays, who gets laid, and who gets the blame.

My transformation, however, was not from bottom to top, but from bottom to bottom: from my wretched emotional submission to my blessed sexual submission. This is the story of my switch—and of paying its price. Very expensive. Priceless.

The SURRENDER

THE HOLY FUCK

> This pleasure is such that nothing can interfere with it, and the object that serves it cannot, in savoring it, fail to be transported to the third heaven. No other is as good, no other can satisfy as fully both of the individuals who indulge in it, and those who have experienced it can revert to other things only with difficulty.
>
> —DONATIEN DE SADE

His was first. In my ass.

I don't know the exact length, but it's definitely too big—just right. Of medium width, neither too slender nor too thick. Beautiful. My ass, tiny, a teenage boy's, tight, and tightly wound. Twenty-five years of winding as a ballet dancer. Since age four, the age when I first declared war on my daddy. Turning out the legs from the hips just winds up that pelvic floor like a corkscrew. I worked my gut all my life standing at that ballet barre. Now it is being unworked.

His cock, my ass, unwinding. Divine.

As he enters me I let go, millimeter by millimeter, of the tensing, pulling, tightening, gripping. I am addicted to extreme physical endurance, the marathon of uncoiling intensity. I release my muscles, my tendons, my flesh, my anger, my ego, my rules, my censors, my parents, my cells, my life. At the same time I pull and suck and draw him inward. Opening out and sucking in, one thing.

Bliss, I learned from being sodomized, is an experience of eternity in a moment of real time. Sodomy is the ultimate sexual act of trust. I mean you could really get hurt—if you resist. But pushing past that fear, by passing through it, literally, ah the joy that lies on the other side of convention. The peace that is past the pain. Going past the pain is key. Once absorbed, it is neutralized and allows for transformation. Pleasure alone is mere temporary indulgence, a subtle distraction, an anesthetization while on the path to something higher, deeper, lower. Eternity lies far, far beyond pleasure. And beyond pain. The edge of my ass is the sexual event horizon, the boundary to that beyond from which there is no escape. Not for me, anyway.

I am an atheist, by inheritance. I came to know God experientially, from being fucked in the ass—over and over and over again. I am a slow learner—and a gluttonous hedonist. I am serious. Very serious. And I was even more surprised than you are now by this curiously rude awakening to a mystic state. There it was: God's big surprise, His subtle humor and potent presence, manifested in my ass—well, it sure is one way to get a skeptic's attention.

Anal sex is about cooperation. Cooperation in an endeavor of aristocratic politics, involving rigid hierarchies, feudal positions, and monarchist attitudes. One is in charge, the other obedient. Entirely in charge, entirely obedient. There is no democratic, affirmative-action safety net swinging below ass-fuckers. But they'd best be of firm action, very firm. You can't half-ass butt-fuck. It would be a travesty. There are no understudies, no backups, for anal Cirque du Soleil. It's a high-wire act—all the way up.

The truth always shows itself with the ass. A cock in an ass operates like the arrow on a lie-detector test. The ass doesn't know how to lie, it can't lie: it hurts, physically, if you lie. The pussy, on the other hand, can lie at the mere entry of a dick in the room—does so all the time. Pussies are designed to fool men with their beckoning waters, ready opening, and angry owners.

I've learned so much, maybe the thing of most importance, from getting fucked in the ass—how to surrender. All I learned from the other hole was how to feel used and abandoned.

My pussy proposes the question; my ass answers. Ass-fucking is the event in which Rainer Maria Rilke's hallowed dictum to "live the question" is, in fact, finally embodied. Anal penetration resolves the dilemma of duality that is introduced and magnified by vaginal penetration. Ass-fucking transcends all opposites, all conflicts—positive and negative, good and bad, high and low, shallow and deep, pleasure and pain, love and death—and unifies them, renders all one. This, for me, is therefore The Act. Butt-fucking offers spiritual resolution. Who knew?

If I were asked to choose for the rest of my life only one place of penetration, I would choose my ass. My pussy has been too wounded by false expectations and uninvited entries, by movements too selfish, too shallow, too fast, or too unconscious. My ass, knowing only him, knows only bliss. The penetration is deeper, more profound; it rides the edge of sanity. The direct path through my bowels to God has become clear, has been cleared.

Norman Mailer sees the sexual routes in reverse: "So that was how I finally made love to her, a minute for one, a minute for the other, a raid on the Devil and a trip back to the Lord." But Mailer is a man, a perpetrator, a penetrator, not a recipient, not a submissive. He hasn't been, I assume, in my compromising position.

My yearning is so large, so gaping, so cavernous, so deep, so long, so wide, so old and so young, so very young, that only a big cock buried deep in my ass has ever filled it. He is that cock. The cock who saved me. He is my answer to every man who came before him. My revenge.

I see his cock as a therapeutic instrument. Surely only God could have thought of such a cure for my bottomless wound—the wound of the woman whose daddy didn't love her enough. Perhaps the wound is not psychological in source at all, but truly the space inside that yearns for God. Perhaps it is merely the yearning of a woman who thinks she cannot have Him. A woman whose daddy told her long ago that there is no God.

But I want God.

Getting fucked in the ass gives me hope. Despair hasn't got a chance when his cock is in my ass, making room for God. He opened up my ass and with that first thrust he broke my denial of God, broke my shame, and exposed it to the light. The yearning is no longer hidden; now it has a name.

∞

This is the backstory of a love story. A backstory that is the whole story. A second hole story, to be entirely accurate. Love from inside my backside. Colette declared that you couldn't write about love while in its heady hold, as if only love lost resonates. No hindsight for me in this great love but rather behind-sight—cited from the eye of my behind. This is a book where the front matter is brief and the end matter is all. After all, my end does matter. When you've been ass-fucked as much as I have, things get both very philosophical and very silly very quickly. My brain has been rocked along with my guts.

Having a cock in her ass really gives a woman focus. Receptivity becomes activity, not passivity. There's just a whole lot to do. His cock pierces my yang—my desire to know, control, understand, and analyze—and forces my yin—my openness, my vulnerability—to the surface. I cannot do this alone, voluntarily. I must be forced.

He fucks me into my femininity. As a liberated woman, it is the only way I can go there and retain my dignity. Turned over, ass in the air, I have little choice but to succumb and lose my head. This is how I can have an experience my intellect would never allow, a betrayal to Olive Schreiner, Margaret Sanger, and Betty Friedan, and an affront, from the rear, to many modern "feminists." Oh, but once there, there is no going back—not to control, not to being on top, not to men more feminine than me. This is simply how my liberation manifested itself. Emancipation through the back door would never be, for any rational woman, a choice. It can only happen as a gift. A surprise. A big surprise.

This story is about my coming to experience—and sometimes understand—terms that allude to spiritual endeavor. I have learned more of their meaning and power through being sodomized than through any other teaching.

Anal sex is, for me, a literary event. The words first started flowing while he was actually buried deep in my ass. His pen to my paper. His marker to my blotter. His rocket to my moon. Funny where one derives inspiration. Or how one gets the message.

I knew after my initiation that I must write it all down. To keep track, bear witness to myself, to him, to the harmonic energy we generated. Enough to burn holes through the parameters of my existing world. Enough for the word God to take on meaning. Enough for gratitude to flow like water.

I didn't want, afterward, just a memory. Memory would inevitably mar the truth with the vanity of nostalgia and the self-pity of lost desire. I wanted documentation, like a police log, which noted at the time—or moments later, an hour at most—the details of the crime, the crime of breaking and entering my ass, my heart. This record would say: this did happen, this did indeed come to pass in my own life, under my own watch.

Besides, if I didn't write it all down, no one would ever believe it—least of all me. I didn't believe it two hours after he left my bed. So I wrote it all down to make it last longer. To make it real. Words seemed the only way to mark the spot, to preserve my transitory experience of eternity. This is a testamentary document. Do not miss the message, distracted by the profanity of the act.

I am, you see, a woman who has been in search of surrender my whole life—to find something, someone, to whom I could subsume my ego, my will, my miserable mortality. I tried various religions and various men. I even tried a religious man. And then he found me, the agnostic who demanded my submission.

"Bend over," he'd say, gently, firmly. I can hear it now—echoing in the bowels of my being.

Ass-fucking is the great anti-romantic gesture—unless of course, like me, your idea of romance begins on your knees with your face in a pillow. Poetry, flowers, and promises till-death-do-us-part have no place in the backland. Ass-entry involves the hard edge of truth, not the soft folds of sentimentality inherent in romantic love. But butt-fucking is more intimate than pussy-fucking. You risk showing your shit, as metaphor and reality. You let a man into your bowels—your deepest space, the space that all of your life you are taught to ignore, hide, keep quiet about—and consciousness is born. Who needs diamonds, pearls, and furs? Those who've never been where I have been. The promised land, the Kingdom.

If you can let a man ass-fuck you—and only the truly sensitive lover should have that privilege—you will learn to trust not only him but yourself, totally out of control. And beyond control lies God.

Humiliation is my greatest devil, but when the eye of my terror is entered, I experience my fear as unfounded. It is through this physical surrender, this forbidden pathway, that I have found my self, my voice, my spirit, my courage—and the cackle of the crone. This is no feminist treatise about equality. This is the truth about the beauty of submission. The power in submission. To me, you see, I have happened upon the great cosmic joke, God's supreme irony.

Enter the exit. Paradise waits.

BEFORE

THE SEARCH

Finding Paradise began decades ago with my search for God. I've been looking for Him since I was five, when my family moved to the Bible Belt. Everyone there seemed to know God personally except me. I asked my father. He was right about everything. "No, there is no God," he explained. "That is for people who need it. We don't."

But I did. Everyone at school was God-fearing and churchgoing. Could they all be wrong, and their parents, too? I was certified at birth an atheist. The deed was done. I figured that I could break the big news to all my classmates that God didn't exist, or I could investigate God on my own, just in case they were right about Him.

Now I think that one can come to believe in two ways. Either you are indoctrinated by your family and that belief stays with you for life, despite rebellion or evidence to the contrary; or you have an actual experience of God that is powerful enough to contradict your original indoctrination. So I assumed a difficult identity: that of the atheist who longs to believe—but can't. Preordained doubt always left me yearning for a God who couldn't exist. The Conflict was born, the Search began.

∽

The previous year, at age four, I had begun ballet classes. This simple, once-a-week affair developed over the course of the next two decades into a ten-year professional career in one of the world's best dance companies. My mother's original intention, however, was simply to give me a physical workout to encourage my nonexistent appetite, and to keep me out of team sports that used balls: as a child, I had an outright terror of balls of any size heading in my direction. Ballet had no balls, and thus my fears were allayed. I concentrated instead on cute outfits, red ballet slippers, and highly controlled movements.

It was in the world of ballet that my investigation of God found its greatest laboratory. Quite simply, all the best dancers believed in God—each and every one. I conducted several private surveys over the years, and continued my God-watch right through my professional career, where the evidence was the strongest. In ballet school, around 60 to 70 percent of the young ladies believed in God; among those who had crossed the hurdle and become one of the chosen few for the company, the percentage rose to about 95 percent. I deduced that the key to these dancers' superiority lay in their ability to believe. They retained faith when things went badly. When I had a bad class, I was bad, which then led to more bad classes. When they had a bad class, they believed it was a "lesson," "God's will," a blip on the screen, and proceeded to have a good class next time and therefore improve in a steady and predictable

manner. Being an atheist, I had no one to blame; self-doubt blos-
somed in proportion to my bad classes.

After ten years of this kind of training, even a good class looked
bad to me; I had perfected not only my pliés but my ability to criti-
cize myself. I sure wished I could put those bad classes on God like
the other girls—what a relief it would have been. But they were living under an "illusion," while I held up the banner of truth, and so I
soldiered on, a martyr to my atheism. God, I was jealous. Not of
their dancing—of their faith.

My anxiety about this haunting intangible found a productive
outlet when, at age eleven, I taught myself to crochet from a book.
My mother knitted and had taught me the two-needle knit-one-purl-
one routine, but there was always the possibility of a lost stitch, discovered too late to correct. The risk of this appalled me. With
crocheting, however, there were not only far more possibilities for
patterns but there was also no way to lose a stitch.

I began with scarves and berets and graduated to ponchos, turtle-
neck sweaters, bags of every size, lacy blouses with ruffles, ties for
men, bedspreads, and intricate doilies made with very fine sparkling
thread. All those stitches, all that yarn and mercerized cotton, all
those pastel colors, in and out, up and around, winding and unwinding, knot after knot. I was fast, I was good, I was compulsive,
and I was relentless with my hook and thread—everyone in my family wore some strange woolly item I had made for them. I always
had several projects going simultaneously, so my hands never
rested.

Stitchery, I see now, was a perfect repository for my ambitious anal tendencies: each article grew in a controlled and foreseeable manner, and was not subject to the irrational chaos of my existential anxieties. I crocheted my way right through adolescence while sewing ribbons on my toe shoes and attempting to emulate the ethereal faith of my peers.

I believe now that dancing is about two things: good behavior and faith made visible. For me the first was easy, the second impossible—hence more desirable. Being a dancer was my earliest, and perhaps most earnest, attempt to have faith. But it was like trying to be a nun without believing in God. I had effort in abundance, but I could not will faith.

Denying myself food all day long while dancing all day long seemed a good place to begin trying, however. At least I was exercising some self-control, making sure that my body would be as svelte as those belonging to the believing girls. I could do that part without God. Just don't eat until the evening. It felt good. Powerful. With food—or, rather, without food—I could compete with the believers. Why, I could even be thinner than a few of them. I learned early how to transcend pain, deny pain: the bloody toes and strained tendons, the horrid loneliness of being an atheist. Very useful. If I could deny enough, I reasoned, perhaps I could even deny my denial of God.

I became a professional dancer at age seventeen and began performing in public eight times a week. It was then that I started crossing myself before going onstage. I had seen the best dancer in all the world do this, and I thought perhaps this was her secret. So I tried it, in the wings, alone, unseen, before an entrance. It was like performing one more step in the ballet. I wanted it to mean something. And it did. Though it did not bring God into my consciousness, it did demonstrate my belief that ritual was the way to invoke Him, in the unlikely event that He should ever be willing to take me on.

On tour in Paris one summer, I started collecting rosaries from the antique stores on the Boulevard St. Germain—old ones, with chips in the mother-of-pearl. I figured that if they were old and European they would already be suffused by the faith of previous believers and thus, despite my miserable Darwinism, some of their faith might rub off on me. I wore one as a necklace for a while, though I was told it was sacrilege. No matter, I needed that rosary around my neck, massaging its history into my heathen skin.

The rosaries led me to the saints. By age eighteen, I was reading voraciously about them all—Francis, Thomas, Jerome, the two Teresas—but I then honed in on the women who starved, who bled, who beat themselves with birch branches, who licked the oozing wounds of lepers, who woke up screaming in the middle of the night, pierced by God's love. This was really interesting stuff. I briefly entertained the idea of switching professions from ballet dancing—already rather nunlike in its dedications—to being a saint. Certainly nothing seemed more worthwhile, and sainthood appeared to demand the disciplines with which I already had substantial experience: self-control and self-denial. Just how much pain and suffering could I endure, could I choose, could I cause for my-self? Testing my strength in this way sounded immensely attractive.

But after considerable consideration, I reconsidered: becoming a saint would entail even more pain than I could imagine. And what if one suffered all that pain and still didn't see God, still didn't have that mystical union? The risk was very high indeed. Besides, I didn't want to suffer just to suffer. Dancing had taught me about pain for gain, pain for beauty. Pain for pain was self-indulgent, whereas my youthful masochism was both ambitious and realistic. Saint Teresa of Avila would have no competition from me.

Instead, I would stick to dancing and continue plunging my toes into the beautiful, tight, shiny sheaths called pointe shoes. And there was the miracle, made manifest daily on my very own feet. De-spite blistered and bloody evidence to the contrary, my feet didn't hurt at all while ensconced in the shoes, while dancing. They only hurt when the shoes came off, when my foot was released from its satin prison. This curious experience, the ironic marriage of physi-cal discomfort and euphoria, taught me the power of transcen-dence. My pink pointe shoes became my fetishistic ally, my crown of thorns, my bed of nails. I adored my toe shoes.

Alongside my saint obsession, I developed a passion for reading. This passion, I came to believe, detracted from my ultimate success as a dancer by luring me from the circumscribed, nonverbal world of movement to the limitless plains of thought. The Book Phase in-cluded: Simone Weil (beyond my scope to emulate); Nietzsche (Thus Spake he to me); Henry Miller (the romance of poverty in

Paris!); D. H. Lawrence (John Thomas and Lady Jane); Anaïs Nin (sexual liberation between the sheets and on the page—in Paris); Freud (incest is best—or at least inevitable); Thomas Mann (the poetic profundity of X-rays); Henry James (I *am* Isabel Archer, living in the wrong era, in the wrong wardrobe); Virginia Woolf (diary after diary right into the river); Erich Fromm; Eric Hoffer; Ernest Becker (*The Denial of Death*, every page underlined in red); and Søren Kierkegaard (seven tomes in a row, with voluminous notes on either legal pads or index cards . . . I loved Kierkegaard).

These books and their revelations constituted my secret life until I was nearly twenty. Then I lost my virginity. And although my deepest interests have perhaps never changed, they immediately became irrevocably diverted to deriving answers—dancing had presented all the questions—from experience, not only books.

But while all this reading and searching for external connection went on in the early morning and late at night, my deepest allegiance and dependence belonged elsewhere during the day: on the walls of the dance studio, where I could not escape my savage self.

MY MIRROR, MY MASTER

Ballet dancing is learned in front of a mirror. Hours and hours and hours and hours in front of a mirror. As a little girl, as a serious student, and then as a professional adult in both classes and rehearsals, I learned that every arch of the foot, every glance of the eye, every angle of the arm, every turn of the leg, every smile, every grimace, every strain is simultaneously performed and witnessed by one's self, that nebulous entity called consciousness. One becomes both subject and object.

I have calculated that in twenty-five years of dancing I spent approximately eighteen hundred hours performing in front of a live audience—and eighteen thousand hours practicing in front of the huge floor-to-ceiling mirrors that are a principal feature of every dance studio. This relentless and intense daily exposure has an acute effect on one's so-called self-image. Contrary to popular supposition, it is not narcissism or vanity that is fostered by so much time spent scrutinizing oneself. Quite the opposite. We watch ourselves with eyes trained to be critical, competitive, and comparative. Yes, every now and then, the view is pleasing, beautiful, something worth looking at. But far more often it is the image of an imperfection—of body, of line, of face, of outfit, of movement. Frequently, this single flaw actually seems to obliterate all one's efforts, even one's entire existence.

The mirror shows the impossibility of perfection. And thus a curious intimacy was born: I was constantly shaping, changing, improving, and restyling myself, while the mirror—cold and constant—sat in judgment, like God. The mirror was now jailer and savior, the source of self-contempt and yet the only source of affirmation. I was humbled before the mighty looking glass with its illusion of three dimensions in two. I submitted completely. While God felt distant, the authority of the mirror over me felt absolute.

I eventually realized that, like Dorian Gray, I had relinquished my entire perception of myself to my reflection. The troublesome result of this submission to what I saw—me, but flipped—was that once onstage, where the orchestra pit and black hole of an audience replaced my own image in the mirror, I could not even feel my body move. I existed solely in the mirror; onstage I was my own shadow, a vapor. Only the next morning, back at the barre, could I find myself in the mirror and once again confirm my existence.

At the age of twenty-three, while still dancing, I attempted to marry God. It was all very sudden. His father was a minister and he was a believer, and so my searching, frustrated atheist self tried to get religion the only way she could: by marrying into the family. My husband was the first man who reflected back to me an image of myself preferable to the one in the mirror. Thus I quickly transferred my dependence to his point of view. Now I existed, but differently. He adored what he saw and told me all about it; it was a lovely thing. Once again, I had good reason to suspect that I had an existence.

As time went on, however, he became far less reliable to show me to myself on a daily basis. He was an acquisitive man of many artistic passions, and others eventually took my place. My reflection became blurred; too many fingerprints upon the once-clear looking glass. Smeared, reduced to a smudge in his mind, I found myself dancing numbly in the black hole one more time. God had turned off the spotlight.

Where am I? I cannot see. I cannot feel. I must not be.

SEX HISTORY

I had my first orgasm, alone, at age sixteen, after going to a French porn movie called *Exhibition* at an Upper East Side art house in New York City with an equally curious girlfriend. Despite the legitimate location, this was my first moviegoing experience where my feet stuck to the floor in front of my seat; this was rather disturbing to my virgin soul.

While watching the woman in this movie masturbate, however, I realized that I had simply not persisted long enough with my own explorations to get to the big bang. I went straight home after the movie and imitated my new mentor, with instant results. Thus began my long and secret career as an aspiring porn star.

I continued practicing for my debut, but saw no reason to employ a man for the job. A year later, a geeky young boy put his tongue down my throat at a party while pressing something very hard up against my belly. This confirmed my suspicions. Men were gross.

Sometime later, a handsome womanizer who knew I was a virgin persisted in pursuing me, and managed to change all these negative feelings. He was famous, strong, charismatic, and sexy as hell. Don Juan. After much resistance, which amused him, I allowed him in. Excitement, pressure, a pool of blood, and awakening.

I had never seen an erect penis before. Totally shocking. But once he started in on me, I got over it. He dominated me—physically, completely—and it was the most thrilling thing that had ever happened to me. I don't believe, however, that I ever had an orgasm with him: I was too excited. And totally in love with him. He suggested a world beyond my own.

I fell in love for two years although the affair lasted less than three months. Looking back, I now realize that his first sexual comment to me was, "You have a great ass." Must have been my fate, even then. But I didn't know it for many years. I look good, from the back.

After I lost my virginity, my pussy became a place of great interest to me. I had not realized until then that that hidden hole below my waist was the entrance to my heart. Others came to the now-opened gate, and I proceeded to have what everyone else seemed to be having: consecutive monogamous relationships of varying lengths. It never occurred to me that you didn't have to become monogamous the moment a guy put his tongue in your mouth. That's just the way it was—sealed with saliva—and I didn't have enough experience to think that I might have a choice in the matter. The second and third boyfriends—both "nice" and "appropriate" young men—introduced me to orgasms through oral sex and I became hooked on that, on their tongues, but not so much on them. The intercourse that followed just seemed like their part of the deal. And there were a few more boyfriends after them. Same thing.

The only time I had sex that was not defined by monogamy was with a stagehand I met in a bar. Long blond hair, gruff language, tattoos. I was having a drink with friends one night when he turned to me and whispered, "I want you to sit on my face."

"Excuse me?" I said. I had no idea what he was talking about. He thought I must be joking, but I wasn't. So he explained. I had another vodka, left the bar with him, and sat on his face. I'd never done that before. He had big hands that handled me like meat, prime. It was my second taste of being with a man who was "wrong" for me, a man with whom I knew there would be no "relationship." Fucking him, I felt the fantastic power of a completely other being crashing into mine. I could not lose myself with a peer, only with a man who was impossible.

But then I fell deeply, suddenly, and totally in love with the man who became my husband—it was like being hit with a cement block on the head, *crash*, and there I was at the altar—and bad boys were banished. It never even occurred to me to have an affair while I was married. I loved him too much, it was unthinkable.

He was my fate, my husband. But I had thought that meant my ending, my final destination, when, in fact, he was my beginning, my wretched beginning. God, that hurt. The profound disillusionment of having the great love of my life founder on the rocky road of reality was a blow too great for my own consciousness to bear, much less comprehend.

After ten years I left my husband. He couldn't see me any longer; and he never even knew I had an asshole. I had retired from dancing some years earlier because of a hip injury that had first surfaced six months into my marriage. Funny, that: life's wicked signposts. A friend says hips represent where you hold trust in your body. Hokum? Maybe. Either way, both my right hip joint and my trust were shot.

I became intolerable both to myself and my husband. A wailing banshee, a celibate nymphomaniac with a suitcase of resentments and matching lingerie. I listed fifty-two of the former and left with the latter. Freedom. Fear.

THE MASSEUR

This bed thy centre is, these walls thy sphere.

—JOHN DONNE

My first affair began a week after the end of my marriage. Amazing what two phone calls can precipitate: one ended a ten-year relationship, and the other booked a one-hour massage that began the rest of my life.

The adorable masseur. I had already had two massages from him for my wounded hip, and I'd held my breath to conceal my desire: I was still married. But by the next massage I wasn't, and I took my first bold step. I could tell that he was too professional to make an overture, so I decided it was up to me. I planned beforehand that if (ha!) I was aroused again, I would say something by the end of the session—but what? I didn't want to embarrass myself; the risk was high.

At the end of that third massage, dripping with a decade of

sublimated desire, I asked him in a general kind of way, "Do your clients ever get aroused?"

"Yeah," he ventured, and got up from a chair on the other side of the room to come back to the table where I was lying. "But I just let it be." He was young and handsome, with big blue eyes and soft full lips, but this was not the source of my attraction. It was those magic hands. He placed one below my throat and I lost all decency and self-control. He did not retreat but slid his hand under the sheet. In the next few hours, I learned about how his mouth and tongue held the same magic current as his hands, and I thought I would die from the pleasure he gave me. It was a dream of pleasure, of love—yes, love, physical love. And no fucking, just sucking.

When he left I was dazed: never had I been so receptive. My clit had come out of hibernation, no longer hiding, no longer scared, but reaching out, reaching for direct contact with heaven. For the first time, I was in submission to my own orgasms, trying only to survive the contractions, to stay conscious despite annihilating pleasure. I knew right then that my decision to leave my marriage and break those vows taken before God was worth it. Worth it all for those two hours. I was sure, of course, that it would not happen again. Why would I be so blessed when I also felt so guilty? Guilt, pleasure, and the impossible man: the ingredients of sexual ecstasy were becoming apparent.

I waited the requisite week, counting the days, and called for another massage, expecting nothing, wanting everything. I jumped when the doorbell rang: bathed, perfumed, and obsessed. Again it happened. Again, and again, and again.

One day he suggested a couple of rules—he'd been thinking, like me, about how to make this thing happen when it shouldn't happen. He didn't play with clients: I was the first, so keep it quiet, very quiet. Of course. The other rule: no intercourse. No problem. "We're just going to play," he explained, and I came to understand just what playing really was. Fucking wasn't so interesting to me, anyway. At best it was a return offering for receiving a good licking. Now licking was the sole activity. And he never, ever, in all the time I knew him, took off his shoes. His shoes became our mutual marker that we were still within our limits of decency. Sort of.

He presented me with the first sex I'd ever had that I thought about in words, that I wanted to describe and preserve in words. And so the scribbling began. Every time he came, and left, I went straight to my notebook and wrote it all down. I was experiencing an impossible pleasure, and having it on paper would prove that the impossible existed.

I knew something profound had happened to me: I had shifted from being my small, hurt, wounded, and unhappy self to being a conduit of a pleasure that was far greater than myself, a pleasure that I did not own, but that I could feel. And I could not experience this in silence. I had to tell some unknown, undefined audience. Perhaps that audience was really me, my unbelieving atheist self being told by my transformed sexual self about hope.

He kisses my belly, inside my thighs, my pubic hair. Eventually with a very soft, very gentle tongue, contact is made with my pussy, my clit. My eyes open. I see his lovely eyes, looking at me, mouth buried in my cunt. My knees drop open 180 degrees, my feet press on the sides of his chest, my pussy is pushed into his mouth, contact, contact, contact. He is there a long time. I have many small, very intense orgasms. He moves his tongue and mouth quickly side to side, then stops on the tip, on my center, a tiny pinpoint where my whole being of emotion, power, and love are centered. Legs and belly convulse, contract, vibrate. Through these releases I know it's not over, not finished. Possessed, I explode. My torso rises off the table over and over, his tongue works furiously, my legs are all over, my arms flailing. I am crying, whimpering, never before so conscious of tears of joy, that someone had been so kind to me.

Every time I called, the pleasure was given and received. His tongue held close and soft and fast on my clitoris became the center of the world. And fingers everywhere—fingers on my clit, fingers in my pussy, fingers up my ass—how many tendrils can one man have? I stopped tipping him. But I did buy a series of ten massages at a reduced rate. He insisted, for his own moral welfare (and perhaps mine), that he always give me a massage—although on more than one occasion the massage came after we did.

I was surprised at how much I liked sucking his cock. It was because he had shown me love first, and filled with gratitude, I headed down. I gave this guy the first good blow job I had ever given, one that came from my guts and brought tears into my eyes. It was the first time I was that grateful to a man.

We never saw each other outside of the room in my apartment. We stayed in the bedroom, only going to the kitchen for liquids and the bathroom for rinses. The bedroom was the world. No dinners, no dates, only phone calls to make an appointment. Because my damaged hip had ended my dance career, the massages were paid for by insurance. Insurance for the resurrection of my deeply injured sexual desire.

I was obsessed with my masseur. I tried to fill the time between sessions, wondering, Did I live to see him, or did I see him so I could live? I learned with him that I am most alive, most observant, and most intelligent when sexually engaged. And I experienced for the first time the intense beauty of having a time and place for a lover where sexual pleasure is the mutual purpose, the only conscious intent. After all, you never know where a dinner date is going to end up. So often the conversation runs amok and preempts the possibility of sex afterwards. I like to know when I'm going to have sex—it's too important to leave to chance.

Boundaries around the erotic ... my theory grew wings. A room, a bed, two bodies, music, no intrusions. This was the life I wanted to explore and did—once a week for over a year. "The frame is a border hermetically sealing-off the object, so that all you are experiencing, all that matters, is within that border," wrote Joseph Campbell. "It is a sacred field, and you become pure subject for a pure object." Ugliness, I realized, only enters my love life when real life does. Cars, calls, bills, mortgages, food, family, schedules, money—these are the subjects of controversy and control, and they destroy the erotic bond.

Did he love me? Did he fantasize about me? Did he dream of marrying me? Did he wonder if I had other men and hate it? Did I infiltrate all his waking moments? Did he wonder what our kids might look like? If mental obsession is the evidence of love, I don't think he was in love with me.

But he loved me in the time we were together. Did he focus all his attention on me? Was he gentle and nasty and charming and completely devoted to multiplying my pleasures? Oh yes, he loved me all right. And this kind of love became the kind I wanted. I began distrusting mental men, talking men, and love's verbal declarations. One cannot love by words alone. I had tried that. Giving and receiving words of love, however witty or Shakespearean, is a ruse propounded by poets with inept dicks. One loves by act. Language can clarify and explain and amuse, but it cannot change your being. Experience can.

Sure, I was in love with him. Until I wasn't. I don't believe love is only real when it endures for many years and is marked by the ring of marriage. My wedding ring had only confined me, robbing me, eventually, of freedom and love alike. Love, for me, exists only in a moment of choice in a moment of time: there is no other manifestation except for the one available right now. Repeating those moments is the key.

But the masseur was not real, I decided. He was only my transient sexual angel who kept reappearing with his heavenly message in my bedroom at preappointed hours. Perhaps, I thought, deep in my unexamined soul, I really am a conventional girl who simply got thrown out of orbit, and a boyfriend is what I need. Perhaps the masses knew something I didn't about men and women and love and sex. So I also tried dating. Six weeks per male, quick to sex, oral, but every time they fucked me I felt fucked over and fired them, one by one. They'd get in, get off, roll over, and I'd feel used and underpaid.

So I kept calling the masseur—whom I paid. It was a better deal.

Disappointment is a great teacher—if one survives the lacerations to one's romantic ideal. After my marriage ended I was willing, open, and angry, and nothing that others did or "society" suggested in terms of conducting relationships necessarily held any merit for me. Everything I knew hadn't worked, so I was free to try anything. Most of all, I had valuable firsthand experience that "relationships" that exist in "real life" sooner or later lose their erotic excitement. Not a particularly original notion, but one I now owned. At the same time, being a dreamer, I was adamant that there had to be another way. All was now backwards to me: fuck love and love sucking.

I was discovering that while the theatrical stage left me numb and afraid and invisible, the sexual stage brought out a spontaneous theatricality and confidence that I knew was my truest self—or at least the one that amused me most. So, like a sexual scientist, I set out to test my theories, to adjust them as needed, and to formulate new ones as they evolved. I had already lost everything, so I had nothing to lose. Thus I vacillated between experiments in the nightmare of attachment with nice-nice sex and the thrill of naughty sex without attachment—take your Tantra and shove it up your yoni.

There were only two rules that governed my behavior. One was relentlessly safe sex—I became the Queen of Condoms. The second was the importance of quality control. If the sex isn't awesome, or at least fascinating, get out, stop, shift gears, and change direction with minimum discussion. There were, as a result, plenty of discarded bodies floating in the moat around my castle, but the drawbridge was always down, inviting new specimens into my laboratory. They came in droves.

NEW YEAR'S EVE

A year later. A petite, Pre-Raphaelite redheaded dancer kept flirting with me at the gym where I exercised. She could tell I was a dancer, too: lean, hard-bodied, physically intense. I had never been with a woman, though I had thought about it plenty. The reality seemed far, far away. It wasn't quite as far as I had thought. She had been trying, she told me, to get this Young Man, who also worked out at the gym occasionally, to have sex with her, but had yet to succeed. She was recently out of a seven-year live-in disappointment. Heroin, lies, other women. Her mental masochism, like mine, needed a rest.

One day, I was at the gym in a corner stretching on a mat when I saw the Young Man nearby, resting between exercises. I had hardly ever noticed him before. He was self-effacing, quiet, and ventured carefully. Sitting, stretching over my toes, I asked him for a push on my back. It was not a sexual overture; I wanted a push. I got one.

His hands touched the middle of my back, moved up and down, pressing my tightness, and I released—even moaned a little. We said nothing. Just his firm fingers pushing deeply, consciously, up and down my back. Time stood still until he took his hands away and I lifted my head, flushed and clear-eyed, as if I'd just come.

We looked at each other, said nothing, stood, went through a fire-exit door into an empty hallway, and slowly pressed into each other, my back to the wall. No words: just eyes and an electric current with European voltage. So much power in one man's hands. It must, physically, be some kind of vibrational force, a quixotic dance of a million molecules. His touch was very strong, very unafraid, and yet so tender. And humble. My belly started contracting involuntarily, and he started trembling through his strength. Yielding, we slid down the wall, stunned. I had never before felt such immediate impact from a man's touch, much less from a stranger. I didn't even know his last name.

It was New Year's Eve that day. The redhead suggested to us both that we spend the midnight hour at her house. Still feeling the effects of his electric field, I agreed. I had no other plans. Neither did he. Would it be him? Her? Both? I didn't know, but I was so willing to find out. And thus fate had her three ways with us.

We convened at the redhead's house at 10:30. Now, this woman knew ambiance like she was born in a harem: red velvet curtains not only on every window but dividing every room; gold fixtures galore; no electric lighting, just candles and incense burning like in a Catholic church; sexy music emanating from unseen speakers; potted palms; naked images of herself in various theatrical guises on the walls; and mirrors, mirrors everywhere—a narcissist's nirvana. I was learning from this woman already, learning about myself, learning what I liked.

After a glass of champagne in crystal flutes at midnight, we ended up on her Persian carpet on some lush pillows watching Fred Astaire in *Top Hat*. The Young Man had never seen it before. He didn't see it that night, either. He and I were the first to touch, relinking from earlier that day. As we grasped hand to hand, she watched like a Cheshire cat, and slowly linked herself, too, to me, hands to legs.

Before long, they had conspired to remove my clothes, mesmerizing my body with touch. Four hands, two faces, male and female, urgent, loving, sexual, groping, they swept me up in waves of love. Gently, they fought over my pussy; he got there first, but she edged him out. The pleasure was illegal. What's wrong with girls with girls? Absolutely nothing. But I wanted to come in his mouth, and in my only move, I pulled his face into me. As I gave him all I had and then some, Fred was still twirling in his top hat on the muted black-and-white screen.

Then the redhead and I stripped him. He allowed it, willing and erect. She and I gathered like good girlfriends around his cock, which was hard, big, and beautiful. Four hands, two mouths. Every few minutes the Young Man raised his head to look down at the scene of angels praying together over his vertical altar. His eyes rolled back in his head, and with a smile and a groan he fell back into his pleasure. But he never came. She commented on his endurance. He said he'd always been that way. She seemed to know a whole lot about cocks and pussies, and I just sucked it all in. He was one of the blessed, she said, a man who can really take a woman on a ride. I found out later for myself just what kind of ride this could be.

Soon after, the redhead announced that she was tired and was going to bed. She showed us a futon that rolled out over the Persian carpet, kissed us both on the forehead, placed two condoms and a bottle of water beside the futon, and disappeared to her own bedroom. She was our fairy godmother, she had felt it between us, she had seen it, and she sanctioned it, even engineered it—despite the fact that she had wanted him. I'd never had a woman do that for me before. I loved the redhead and her house of Freudian mirrors.

And then the blessings really began. Thus far, there had been no fucking that night. Now love poured out of this guy's body like oil. When he entered me, I knew. I just knew. He fucked in love, not frenzy; in tenderness, not anger; in ease, not desperation. What his cock could do for me seemed to be the question he was answering. It did plenty for both of us. Finally, a fuck I liked. A new year, a new world.

I saw him once more, alone, before he went to Europe for two weeks, but I simply didn't have the courage to love him, so I got myself one of those temporary boyfriends—monogamy, weekends away, dinner parties, friends, plans. When the Young Man returned, he called, and I told him I had a boyfriend, I couldn't see him. He was too good to be real, I told myself, so I chose instead a small, jealous man who didn't even like to eat pussy. Why? Self-hatred, lack of faith, and a fear of what is beautiful: divorce can make you nuts. But after the boyfriend snooped in my diary one morning six weeks later and confronted me with questionable evidence—I had kissed the Young Man at the gym and had written it down—I fired him on the spot, my outrage being greater than his. I never saw him again.

So I continued to date some men (dinner) while fucking others (no dinner). I was learning a lot—well, two things anyway. I preferred sex on an empty stomach, and to eat alone with a good book.

MEN

Despite all this emerging knowledge, convention dies hard and I still kept trying out boyfriends—whom I always bitterly resented afterwards for allowing me to entrap myself. But between these misguided debacles there were several amusing forays. The impossibly handsome actor who modeled Jansen bathing suits but whose riveting blue eyes seemed to look into mine only to see their own reflection. It was the first time I witnessed a man's narcissism that was undoubtedly greater than mine—how unbecoming, I thought. His cock was huge and, I suppose, impressive, but it smelled antiseptic and I kept away. The big neighbor who looked like Nicolas Cage was a bit of a jerk, but he fucked so slow that I cried at the beauty, at the sadness. Then there was the other neighbor, the biker. I'd never had a Harley man; never done it before on a Harley, over a Harley. Lost an earring I loved. The cute newspaper boy: the cliché was too good to resist. And he did deliver.

I tried returning to a former boyfriend. Great friend, not a lover. Then there was the guy who held me fast with one arm, his tongue

buried in my mouth, his cock vertical against me while madly wav-
ing with his free hand for a cab to take me away. This has become
my favorite image of male ambivalence.

There was the magician who could produce my jack of hearts
out of sealed cement only seconds after I handed it to him but
who, remarkably for a trickster, couldn't eat pussy to save his life.
Talents vary. One Paul Newman–like prospect found me at Star-
bucks and caught me with his eyes. He could ejaculate, stay hard,
and come again, often three times in row. Remarkable. I wondered if they were three full orgasms, or if he had simply learned
to parse out one big one to impress the girls. He even attempted
boyfriend status, but his patronizing butt-patting made me
crazy. One evening, when he arrived for a date and asked to
hang his clean shirt for the next morning in my closet, I knew
I was done with him. What presumption. Sex does not mean
breakfast.

Happily, the beautiful boys—tall, svelte, toned, thoughtful, loving, full of poetry and music—never considered sleeping over, but
they did not yet know how to fuck, either. I was intrigued by two feet
guys. Sucking, kissing, rubbing my feet in stilettos, they garnered
erections like steel. But was it me or my shoes? I do have some great
shoes. They both had big cocks—about the height of my heels,
strangely enough—dispelling any misconception I might have had
that their fetish was compensatory.

A charming young Frenchman produced the thickest cock I'd
ever seen up close. He knelt above me, shoving this enormous

protrusion toward my mouth, saying "Suck it, suck it," with a strong French accent. It was the size of a corncob. I was terrified. Condoms didn't fit, they kept rolling back to the tip like a bad joke that was very funny. Finally, I rolled one on three inches with much cock to spare and we had a three-inch, fat fuck.

After seriously considering the evidence of my current sexual escapades, I concluded that I did not like intercourse. The Young Man had been a strange exception. Either they were not so big, and I felt little, and the whole event felt feeble: the Princess and the Pea. Or they were so big it hurt and my anger would increase with every thrust until I became the victim of a monstrous rage.

Besides, I almost never had an orgasm from fucking except for the one guy who would direct me to climb on top and "make" myself come. He would just lie there, rigid in body and cock, and I would follow his directive and rub my clit on his pubic bone. But, I thought, this was not coming from intercourse, this was masturbating with a live dildo. I ended up resenting his orders until my only defense, ironically, was *not* to come.

Every man who fucked me risked my contempt—and most earned it. The smart ones stayed away or insisted on friendship, while the arrogant ones plunged in to their enormous satisfaction— and eternal regret. There were also, of course, the romantics, who thought they wanted a woman like me—but they didn't, not really, not once they'd seen my version of romance.

Was I gay and wasting my time with men? I adore beautiful, feminine, bright women: if I was so anti-penetration and so clitorally oriented, maybe they were the way to go. But conquering men—or, rather my resentment of them—has always seemed a far more interesting challenge. I reckon every woman wants a cock between her legs, ultimately. The question is: Does she want one of her own, or can she tolerate one belonging to a man?

SCANTY PANTIES

It is perhaps no surprise, given my theatrical background, that props, costumes, and ceremony became increasingly essential components of my newly expanded private life. My bed became the stage for that intense human drama called sexual interplay. I knew from public performance that artifice, ambiance, and ritual could propel the participant into a state of truth and beauty far more effectively than thoughts or good intentions. In my bedroom, where I exchanged my tutus for corsets, my tiaras and toe shoes for blindfolds and stilettos, the poetic logic was obvious. And crotchless panties fit perfectly (they always do) into the tragicomedy that was now my sex life. This vastly underrated, overlooked undergarment is so rarely celebrated, or even mentioned, that I must digress for just a moment to rectify this enormous oversight.

While the thong has been elevated to a sexual status far beyond its actual utility, the crotchless panty is really where it's at, or at least where my clit is at. I actually—optimistically and sadly—bought my first pair while still married. Black, transparent little nylon bikinis without any crotch between the leg elastics. The moment I saw them—draped over a red silk hanger at a sex store I visited while in Copenhagen on vacation—I got a warm rush. Ah, another Danish souvenir to bring home along with my crotchless Little Mermaid statue. But this lonely item simply ended up gathering dust in the back of my underwear drawer—until found, washed, and resurrected in my new single life, years later. The first time I put them on for a lover was a brave day indeed. But they received a most encouraging reaction. I needed another pair. But where to shop?

Crotchless panties are usually found in sex-toy stores and occasionally, in small supply, at Frederick's of Hollywood, where the variety is also quite limited. Despite their titillating sell, Victoria's Secret stops just short of offering their slutty little panties with crotch slits. But where, after all, is "Victoria's Secret"? It sure isn't at their return address in Ohio. I guess this is where those masters at monitoring the boundary between decency and vulgarity draw the line to maintain their legitimacy. But the sex stores have a different reputation to maintain, and they are well stocked. Costing on average just slightly more than your basic cotton thong but far less than La Perla's little nothings, these crotchless wonders will definitely get you more bang for your buck.

Crotchless panties are actually little works of art, and the art is clearly in the details—or carefully placed lack of detail. They are, in short, pussy-framing devices—hence their great potential for lovers, even going so far as to guide those who are directionally challenged right into the center of the playing field. Contrary to popular assumption, they come in many different styles—each with its own *je ne sais quoi*. I currently own five styles, with a few duplicates of my favorites.

There is the very normal-looking bikini style—mine are deep purple—that upon closer inspection (which is the aim, after all) sport a very nasty little three-inch, black-lace-lined slit in the middle of the crotch that basically forms a glory hole for a searching tongue—or cock. In their apparent innocence, these are in some ways the naughtiest of the assortment—but then again perhaps not . . . There are the transparent black ones that carry the slit concept to infinity: the slit, red-ribbon-rimmed, simply runs from the waistband in front all the way down and around to the waistband in back. These are actually very practical panties, allowing for clit, cunt, and ass access, although with one's legs held together, they appear quite decent.

Then there is my little-girl pair: white with tiny pink roses. These are stylistically quite complex. While they retain the usual waist of a panty, the entire crotch has been excised, leaving only two delectable little elastics traveling between one's legs with zippo in between except one's very own jewelry box. Carefully coiffed pubic hair in front acquires a really lovely triangular frame in this style, and I'm especially charmed by the petite pink bows decorating the crucial junctures where skin and panty meet. Taken as a whole, this truly "crotchless" design is perhaps the most elegant of the bunch, but I'm also fond of a rather amusing pair that has clearly been based on the design of a ballerina's tutu. Sporting a split thong between the legs and a witty little tutulike black gauze ruffle around the waistband, they are quite adorable.

But the very best of all, my favorite, is the Butterfly. I have these in both black and powder pink. These are the most expensive and it is clear why—they have the least fabric of all. These petite, delicate works of art best embody the great irony of this particular garment: they are classy crotchless panties.

G-string style, the upper pubic area is designed and woven in the shape of a spread-eagled butterfly complete with wings sprinkled with beads and shimmering sequins. I just adore glitter, pomp, and circumstance around my pussy—I'd wear red velvet curtains with gold-tasseled tiebacks between my legs if I could. But the real pièce de nonrésistance in these particular panties lies in the two slender elastic straps that connect the lower wings of the butterfly to the center of the thin elastic waistband in the back. Properly placed, alongside the outer pussy lips, they pull up ever so slightly, visually accentuating from the front the beginning of one's slit.

But one day those two little straps slipped—ooh la la!—and demonstrated yet again that accident is the mother of invention. With those elastics placed securely inside, on either side of one's clit and hood, the butterfly soars. Oh my, oh my, oh my—that feels good. And it looks absolutely beyond porn queen, like the summit of high art—like a Modigliani by Mondrian.

To be so framed, positioned, and exposed and then have a lover find his target—well, I could come right now just thinking about it. It seems to me to be, at the very least, respectful to utilize these various crotchless darlings to aid and abet those men whose only object is my clit and whose only reward is my clit.

HOUND SEX

In those first years after my marriage, I discovered that the great antidote to bad fucking—or no fucking—is fantasy, and that fantasy's greatest aide is the Pussy Hound: the man who lives to dive. Every woman should have at least one; it can mend years, even centuries, of patriarchal ramming. Thank heaven, then, that women's liberation has fostered what appears to be an entire generation of this particular man: the male masochist who can now masquerade, legitimately, as the feminist man, the male lesbian. They can be spotted on street corners everywhere. I say grab one, girls, and give him a job!

The masseur had taught me how to make my orgasm, not his, the main event, how to allow oral sex to compete successfully, even override, intercourse. After all, for women, cunnilingus is a much more dependable pleasure. This is a hard lesson for a nice girl to learn, what with so many dicks always demanding attention. Hounds help. And so do crotchless panties. In fact, it is with a headstrong Hound that crotchless panties find their true place.

First as a good girl, then as a married woman who didn't dare imagine having sex with anyone but her husband, I'd had a fairly impoverished fantasy life. But once the masseur came along and became a real-life fantasy, that potent world was cracked open and my desires came tumbling out.

All those unlived scenes told me a lot about myself. There was the rich woman who pays for cunnilingus—and I did pay, cash. There was the trashy girl in six-inch heels and crotchless wonders— "Lick my shoes! Lick them clean!" And then there was the virgin in Victorian white cotton whose rich father pays the "healer" to give her her first orgasm: it is the only way to save her life, for she is, of course, mortally ill. She resists mightily, feigning sleep and frigidity, and comes like a rolling avalanche—brought back from the brink of death by the anonymous roving tongue.

The whore fantasies were prolific and my fee enormous. I found it fascinating that the man who materialized in these heated encounters was more often than not almost physically repugnant to me—a beast-man. Being a sucker for beauty in general, I gave this unexpected scenario a great deal of thought. I concluded that every woman must have a man—real or imaginary—to whom she is a whore, for whom she is a whore. I have always wanted, alas, to be some man's bimbo. I don't mean just acting like a slut or being desired for sex alone, although these are both excellent goals. I mean that the sex is for profit—be it financial or otherwise—more than for physical desire. If a woman is driven by a physical craving, she is vulnerable; with a beast-man, obviously, she retains her power. But that is not the most interesting part.

I also discovered that imaginary sex with a man for gain is incredibly sexy. One's inner whore gets a real workout, so to speak. Selling one's sexuality, by choice, frees a woman's desires from the incriminations, restrictions, and suppressions of good-girlness that proliferate when one is "in love." And thus the paradoxical surprise: love is released as gratitude in great gushes of incredible uncensored sexual energy. With my fantasy beast-men I achieved orgasms that were, finally, entirely guiltless; they were, after all, my job. You see, I have an impeccable work ethic, whereas in matters of the heart I have no idea of my rights, much less their application. When sex becomes my work, I'm home free—cash in hand.

I found that if I allowed these various fantasies to rove uncensored, they would uncover parts of myself that were otherwise entirely hidden. I became particularly interested in the fraction of time that preceded the moment of orgasmic inevitability. What thought, what dynamic, what image would cause that final, magical, loss of control? That was the pivotal moment that seemed to join consciousness to the divine—and more often than not, I found this lofty pathway to be inspired by completely slutty activities (see above—and below). This meeting of the galaxies in the gutter fascinates me still.

I learned, for example, that I often reach the point of inevitability through the inspiration of a dire "last-resort" thought or image that renders me, my pussy, my clit, the most exposed, the most seen, the most helpless. Loss of responsibility—it's-not-my-fault—does it every time.

My OB-GYN fantasy works extremely well: I am the guinea pig, for a fee of five hundred dollars—I really need the money; it's only for the money—for the final semester of classes for the advanced medical students. I am behind a big white sheet, just doing it for the dough, awake, and above it all—this is work. On the other side of the sheet my feet are in stirrups, my thighs are wide, and my pussy is spread for show-and-tell. The doctor teaching the class first uses a pointing rod to direct the ten students to the sites of the female sexual anatomy. Then, naughty doctor, he starts to use his fingers to better explain the details. And all those students, male and female, are gazing intently at my shaved, pink little pussy while I read the *New York Times* Arts & Leisure section on the other side of the sheet, blasé and anonymous, feeling nothing . . . I think.

The final class is devoted to the clit and female sexual excitement, with the doctor suggesting that for thorough knowledge each student get up real close for a single, well-earned lick before their lunch break. By now I am somewhat distracted and wondering why the *Times* doesn't have a horoscope section, and then the good doctor finishes me off, showing all those young men and women just how expert a physician he really is. Now I know my horoscope: it's a "good day," full of "unusual opportunity" with a "tempting offer" for "a lucrative position promising unexpected personal reward."

About anonymity and sex. I find it very shortsighted to dismiss the concept of "anonymous" sex—real or imagined—as "impersonal," and shamefully indicative of one's unresolved "intimacy issues." This is a terrible misunderstanding based on the post-

Freudian world where "individuality" and "self-expression" have been raised to unworthy heights of worthiness that leave one saddled with the heavy burden of "being oneself" at all times. Who can be "themselves" during sex? Not me.

In anonymity lies freedom from oppression—from the personality of one's partner, and from one's own demanding ego. Blindfolds are your friends, concealing your shame and the identity of your all-too-human lover. Anonymous sex is not about avoidance. For me, it is about a kind of harmless grandiosity: when I am anonymous, I exist as something far greater than my particulars. I become an archetype, a myth, a Joseph Campbell goddess spreading my legs for the benefit of all mankind for all time. This imagined generosity brings me the most profound orgasms.

One heroic diver would come over, eat me out, slowly, slowly, daring me not to come. Sometimes I'd last over an hour. How wonderful to be in the position of trying to hold back, of not praying to come. There was one thing he did want, to lick my ass. Okay, I said, go ahead. But he didn't just lick my ass, he fucked my ass with his tongue, very impressive indeed, never had a tongue deeper to date. He never took his clothes off, and he had the good taste to never kiss me on the mouth.

There is risk, however, with the Pussy Hounds. The final fading of my respect has sometimes happened when a man is so eager to suck my pussy that I know he indulges his need to please rather than an actual love of pussy. It's distracting. Intention is all—I can feel it with my clit. It is more important to me that a man love pussy in general than mine in particular. After all, if he likes them as a whole, then mine is a slam dunk. But if a man likes only mine and not all the others, well, I just don't trust him. With this type of man I have learned to guide my orgasm with fantasy, and, like him, play the using game. While he licks furiously, indulging his codependence, I file through my Rolodex of every man I've ever known, all in the audience, erections puncturing the air, watching this one lap at the altar they all still covet. Works every time.

It is my altruism, not my narcissism, that fosters this fantasy. After all, a man can acquire such wisdom at the source of a woman's orgasm: how to slow down, speed up, be consistent, be nonlinear, be persistent, be unpredictable, be patient, be outrageous, be generous, be witty. There is, in fact, nothing of value, philosophically and practically, that he can't learn if he can turn the delta of Venus into the site of Vesuvius.

Most men will lick and suck and drink a pussy—and I'm not complaining. But it is the rare man who does so with his whole consciousness poised on his tongue. It is this awareness that will move a woman; when her consciousness—on her clit—encounters his, orgasm marks their meeting. Ultimately, it is here—or rather, down there—that a man will learn how to be a winner or a loser, with women as in life.

TRINITY

If old-fashioned fucking-for-two remained a minefield for me, fucking-for-three continued to be a delight. The Pre-Raphaelite redhead plotted reunions, and we three got together every month or so with unplanned regularity for over a year. I returned to my New Year's Eve lovers again and again, hungry for love and freedom — a previously impossible duet in my experience. Says Jesus in the Gnostic Gospel of Thomas:

> *When you make the two one, and when you make the inside like the outside and the outside like the inside, and the above like the below, and when you make the male and the female one and the same . . . then you will enter the kingdom.*

One day, I ventured down on the Pre-Raphaelite. First time. Terrified. Curious. I wanted to see her pleasure in order to know my own. She was a genuine redhead. Eating pussy when you are a heterosexual woman is overwhelming. To confront a pussy that close for the first time — you can't ever get that close, at that angle, to your own—is like looking narcissism in the face with a resounding Yes! Profound. Wet.

It can sometimes be so hard to be oneself in one's own sex life. With another woman, a woman's identity receives a brutal jolt: she is me, I am her, her pleasure is mine, mine is hers. The source, the center, the origin of the human race becomes your only view. I bonded with my own sex and learned to love myself. I also developed a new compassion for the male divers. A pussy is a wild and watery landscape of hills and valleys and ravines and mighty holes that suck one in like quicksand. Once in, you cannot escape. Diving is an act of bravery.

The redhead, however, demonstrated less hesitancy, and ate me like a woman who knows how. Naughty, considerate, and relentless. Her fingers felt like tongues, her mouth like a baby's, sucking. I resist men's fingers. Too rough, too big, too fast. My shield goes up, my clit hides. My orgasms with her were long, open, and free.

The next New Year's we three reconvened and she had a surprise for us: her beautiful young Belgian friend who was mourning the loss of her rock-star lover. One-two-three-four, three of one and one of the other. She and me and him . . . and her. I did a striptease to Led Zeppelin, swinging around the luscious green velvet curtains at the door of her boudoir—a kind of *Gone With the Wind*–Vivien-Leigh-Gone-Wild moment.

The Belgian girl was shy, but she didn't shy away. The redhead

and the Young Man looked at each other slyly, and before I knew it
they had lined me and the beautiful Belgian up on the bed side by
side; he devoured my pussy while the redhead ate hers. I looked to
my left, catching eyes and hands with the Belgian. I felt so safe. Later
he and I lay faceup underneath the soft white ass of the kneeling Belgian, our lips close to hers, as we took turns licking her. "Eat her," I
say, and watch him dive and suck and drink pussy, another pussy. It
made me wild with joy. Later we rolled out another futon and slept,
all four, side by side. In the morning I climbed on his hard cock
while the other two watched, the Belgian reaching out and holding
his hand while we fucked for her, for us. Loving and hot . . . like hell
on fire. That was New Year's Day. This was my unmarried life.

The Young Man and I fucked alone as well. But when the redhead
told me she had seduced him without me, I didn't like it—no, not
one bit. It was legal and democratic—the three of us had no rules—
but it felt horrid to be left out of the party. And horrid, in my new-
found sexual bravado, to experience something so shameful as
jealousy. I had never felt this particular pain before, having only
been with faithful men. The three of us met at his place and tried to
talk about what was hurting me.

I was playing with fire all right, but it burned so brightly that I
could not, and would not, acknowledge the warning that had just
come my way. Between all the forbidden ecstasy I was having, I
was still weeping on a regular basis over my marriage, and still

interpreting all grief as emotional weakness. It seemed such an awful bore to be jealous, so bourgeois. Surely I could overcome this feeling with practice, with the right bohemian attitude.

They countered my fear—fear of loss of him, of her, of our magic triangle—by telling me how much they both loved me. I told them that I loved them, too . . . and that I wanted to see them fuck. I put the condom on him and, leaning over his back, guided his cock between her legs and into her. We both looked down on her, the delicate little redhead, as he fucked her, and I saw myself: pale, vulnerable, and pierced. But I was also him, fucking her with a big beautiful cock, riding his back as he pulsed in her, me.

Later I lay on my back and she climbed on top of me, small, white, fragile. Breast to breast, mouth to mouth, we lined up our pussies, redhead and brunette, hers mine, mine hers. Over her, he entered me, six legs atop one another. I looked up at their two faces beaming down on me as he fucked me. I held them both and knew that this was one of the great moments of my life—of being overwhelmed, ensconced in love. He is me is she is he and we are rolling, fucking, oozing, laughing, being.

This layered, fucking sex sandwich became the image for my final theory of us three. He and I deeply connected, with her as our midwife, our buffer, our catalyst, our crazy glue. As Colette observed, "Certain women need women in order to preserve their taste for men." She lightened us, separated us, and spread around the shattering intensity between us. She diminished the terrible anxiety of love.

Several months later, he announced he was leaving town for a job—for months and months, maybe forever. We hastily arranged a rendezvous. After he arrived, she called to suggest we begin without her, she would be late. She knocked just as we finished fucking. We greeted her naked, but she was in red velvet and green silk with freshly cut white baby roses strewn in her hair, like Ophelia.

They told me to just lie there, and relax, as they connected over their prey. He had fingers on my clit, up my pussy, and inside my ass, while she leaned over me, soft, with red, silky hair everywhere, whispering "I love you, I love you, I love you, I love you . . ." The waves started coming and still he continued, still she whispered, caressing my face, "I love you, I love you, I love you . . ." The waves continued, on and on, with orgasms so sweet building to ones less sweet but more intense.

And then it happened. A wave began in my feet and legs, traveled up my belly, my chest, my throat, and my soul burst out the crown of my head. It was the deepest experience of pleasure-love I had ever known—or witnessed. She later explained the technical name was a "Kamikazi-Mega-Hiawatha." That sounded precisely right.

Then he left town. Gone. Gone.

She and I met one sunny afternoon holding each other in her bed, with wandering fingers—but I missed him. Sweet sisters without a cock between us.

MAN OF GOD

The loss felt devastating. Would such joy never be more than momentary? Probably not. My inability to tolerate this knowledge led me into yet another flirtation with God. This time I met him at Home Depot.

I was in a back aisle with a tape measure and a saw trying to cut a seven-foot wood pole in half to use as a curtain rod. The pole kept rolling off the cutting bench, and things were not going well. Finally, as I made the first slice into the wood, my sequined handbag slipped off my shoulder, and the saw went flying out of my hand. He caught it and asked if I would like some help. "Oh yes!" I said, relieved. Well, maybe this was only the carpenter son, but I wasn't going to fuss about generational details at this crucial moment in the lumber aisle. I just knew that he'd saved me.

He was tall, handsome, fair-haired, and soft-spoken. He carried the freshly cut pole to the checkout for me and put it in the trunk of my car. He asked if he could buy me something to eat and we crossed the street to a burger joint. For a four-hour lunch.

How can a single, liberated woman have the indescribable pleasure of illicit sex? No, not with a married man: that's never appealed to me. With a celibate man. Mr. Home Depot was a born-again Christian. *And* a former "sex addict." He said he'd often fucked seven or eight different women in a week! Oh my God! Could this be the perfect man? God and Pervert and Hound all neatly packaged in a six-foot-two Texan. And he was handy, too.

He told me the story of his conversion. Early one October morning on the beach in the Bahamas, after a night of drugs and debauchery, God—unsolicited—had spoken to him, saying: "The time is now." Being a seeker myself, I was jealous. Why hadn't God ever talked to me? I asked if God had spoken out loud—would I have heard Him, too, if I'd been there? But I couldn't get a clear answer on those details. From that day forward, in any case, he had been sober and celibate. This man hadn't had sex for fifteen years. My imagination reeled at the thought of all those lonely erections. Nice, too, that he wasn't newly born-again, but long-term born-again. He knew every book of the Bible, backward, and taught Bible school every week.

The Forbidden married to the Unattainable was my magical aphrodisiac: I realized at that first long lunch that Born Again and I would never, ever have sex, and thus my heart began to open and my pussy to yearn. Once again, the impossible had coalesced before me. He had the biggest hands and feet I'd ever seen. Listening to his story, I began feeling a Christian conversion rapidly coming my way.

He said that it was difficult to find a nice Christian wife—the only way he could legitimately have sex again. I didn't understand; he looked so incredibly eligible. Then he admitted with a shy grin that he liked his women a little slutty—*trashy* was the word he used. Admittedly, I couldn't be a genuine Christian, but I had been practicing slutty and trashy for a few years already. This man's contradictions were as epic as my own.

I asked him just how far could he go sexually before God got mad: "Where is the line?" An hour later, I still hadn't gotten an answer, just a discernible sigh as his tongue hit my clit on the roof of a nearby car park. He had suggested looking at the view. God was now speaking to me, too, and the time *was* now and the view superb. And thus, I, too, died and was born again.

I have never seen a man before or since look at a pussy the way this guy did. I felt penetrated by his gaze alone. He projected an innocent, open-eyed hunger layered with filthy lust and divine desire. It is forever fixed in my mind's eye and, easily recalled, can make me come in a jiffy.

The risk of being caught in public did wonders for Born Again. One afternoon I sucked his cock in a Denny's parking lot, just as the lunch crowd of blue-haired ladies was heading for their Pontiacs. He had a great way of staying calm, cool, and on the lookout above while fucking my mouth furiously below. Jekyll and Hyde, sacred and profane, horny man of God.

Another time he stuck his hard cock through my vertical mail slot, humping my front door, as I sucked him on the other side while neighbors passed behind him in my courtyard. Perhaps this

was a man I could actually date. But shortly afterward he told me
that both Darwin and the Dalai Lama were, in general, wrong
about most things, and my brief hope for a man who combined the
erotic and the spiritual disappeared. When he told me that he didn't
believe in evolution (so I came from a monkey but he didn't?), I
suggested we stop talking entirely and find a nice mail slot through
which to communicate.

This guy name-dropped God like they were buddies, and his
heresies became my self-righteous obsession. Though invited to enter their bliss for a three-way, I simply couldn't override my own intelligence and do it. Witnessing his religious arrogance in all its
shameless glory, however, inspired my own libido to new heights,
and every erection became a tangible victory over his troubled
piety. Dressed in my red stilettos, fishnet stockings, and a thong, I
invited him one night to come into my backyard. Camouflaged in
my bushes, he spied through the bedroom window into the candle-
light as I pranced, stripped, and touched myself. All was quiet but I
could see his hypocrisy harden as his hand moved furiously back
and forth on his cock. Was God watching now as my pussy took
precedence over Him? I couldn't have God myself, so I settled for
treating Him like the competition. In fact, each time Born Again
touched me in public, I felt a kind of religious potency emanating
from my pussy.

I was angry at Born Again for not being who he thought he was.
And who I hoped he was. I wanted him to be for real, a real Man of
God. Once again, I found myself not fucked by God but fucked

over by His apostle. This man's flaws shone all the brighter in the light of my massive expectations and subsequent frustration. I had, you see, loved him. A little. He couldn't win with me, and eventually the games wore out and I ended our X-rated morality play. The Holy Fuck never took place. Perhaps this was how he kept things straight with his buddy.

THE LAST BOYFRIEND

Contrary to appearances, perhaps, I was by now finally beginning to acquire some semblance of romantic discipline. After the disappointment of the truck-driving, gun-toting, sex-addicted Republican Christian, it was time for the Volvo-leasing, pot-smoking, monogamous, left-wing atheist. And a liberal lesson in disappointment.

I refused to mourn for the impossible Young Man and the crazy Christian. So I attempted the possible—a boyfriend with an out-of-control dick—and found this, too, impossible, but in a different way.

There are two types of out-of-control dicks: the first one insatiable, the second merely undisciplined and poorly behaved. I prefer the former, but often found myself with the latter.

In some strange, inexplicable throwback to my premarriage years, I had agreed to be monogamous with this guy after one mad make-out session on my couch on the first date. He asked and I delivered. Perhaps I was having a conventional moment of my own after the transcendent Trinity and the byzantine Christian affair. Naughtiness in the moment was definitely the most fun, the most erotic, but it had a price—the anxiety of impermanence.

Immediately, however, I was reminded of something even worse: the anxiety of permanence. I had hitched myself to a single flawed human being. What was I thinking? Weekly therapy, where I howled bloody murder, kept me "working" on the "relationship" for more than the usual six weeks. For over a year I tried to be his girl-friend, kicking and screaming every step of the way. I even considered Prozac in this last attempt to be "normal" and "conventional." Aren't drugs, after all, how everyone else tolerates monogamy?

I hated being the object of a desperate, controlling passion but felt that it was somehow the morally dutiful stance when the man "loved" me. I was finally cured when I found myself in a fetal position on the floor of my bedroom while the Boyfriend put me on hold for a business call. I had humiliated myself beyond recognition.

What is wrong with me? The wretched question always beckoning my shame, the shame of the little girl who was deemed "overly sensitive." But with the Boyfriend I made progress. I stayed long enough to allow the pain to slice right through my mental masochism and discovered the relief on the other side: my sadism.

I considered the radical possibility that there might be nothing "wrong" with me. Except perhaps choosing guys who adored me, seduced me, and then couldn't control their dicks, and therefore had to control me. I'd protest, get upset, and the discussion would be successfully diverted from their penis to my hysteria. Oh, the myriad insecurities, baffling behaviors, addictions, and possessive outbursts that inhabit the man in search of control. There is only one kind of control that really matters.

My nice-girl martyrdom over, I turned to its heady antidote, the liberation of tyranny. I would no longer accommodate penis problems—whether they were insecurities about length or width, or issues of control lost and not found. If a damaged dick and his owner threatened to raise their heads in my direction, I would simply move out of their reach, and be on my way.

I told the Boyfriend that either we were finished or he could retain me as his mistress—meaning my own mistress. I even wrote down the rules—a parody of a best-selling treatise by a couple of housewives on how to lead a man to the altar. My rules led to slavery instead.

THE REAL RULES

1. See each other a maximum of once a week, except in special circumstances and when it's a mutual decision to do so. A week is defined as Monday through Sunday—hence there can be a Saturday encounter and then a Tuesday encounter but then not until the following Monday, when a new week begins.

2. One encounter is defined as any time spent together with no specific limits on hours, etc.—a late-night horny rendezvous and a weekend away both count equally as one encounter.

3. "Don't ask, don't tell" policy on nonmonogamy issue. But when together, completely together—no procurements, flirtations, etc.

4. Outside issues to be carefully avoided: work, friends, and family.

5. Phone calls are for only two purposes: to plan an encounter, or, if desired, a thank-you follow-up call, postencounter. No long, in-depth discussions of any nature on the phone—not about others, not about our relationship, not about current sports events.

6. Both parties are equally free to initiate the next encounter and the one who calls preferably has an "offer," a "plan." Examples: Be ready at 6 P.M. Friday with an overnight bag, sunglasses, and a jacket; or meet me at Café Lulu at 9 P.M., I'll have no panties on; or movie, dinner, and sex; or a 10 P.M. call—I'm coming over to suck your cock; or pick me up and I'll surprise you; or let's talk and not have sex. . . . Anything and everything can be an encounter, and imagination is all.

7. While together, refinements, additions, and subtractions to rules can be discussed and negotiated, although avoid getting stuck in having the encounters be entirely about the encounters.

8. All these rules, limitations, and boundaries are designed to enable and protect the possibility of fully, deeply, freely exploring the erotic realm and whatever else goes along with it.

9. Can give gifts to each other, but absolutely no obligation in this area.

10. Any amendments to these rules must be very clearly discussed and agreed upon together.

I faxed them over. These rules were a serious, insane attempt to legislate separation, to eliminate all areas of contention, to edit our sex life into our only life. Well, it was worth a try. In truth, #3 was the only rule I really cared about. It legislated hope.

Mistressing worked for a few months. One by one he tested every rule like a naughty boy. He bought me dresses and handbags, and in his arrogance thought he would win me from the competition. But it was too late. Show me an arrogant man, and I'll show you my machete—ah, the legitimized anger of feminism! I had freed myself at last from men whose shit was so deep that I thought it was my own. What I've learned from each relationship is how much emotional pain I'm willing to take. This was the last conventional connection I've had with a man.

This relationship had an unexpected silver lining, however. It goes like this. When I met him, the Boyfriend was deep in therapy with the first shrink of his life. He adored her, praised her, and wanted me to meet her—wanted her approval. I was evidence of how far he had come. Meanwhile I had a shrink, too, who helped me deal with my divorce, but I didn't adore her. I agreed to meet his.

Within a couple of weeks of seeing him, I was already in a state of complete agitation, and so we went to see her together. And I adored her, also. Oh dear.

"Can't I see her, too? You know, separately?" He thought it a fine idea—same mom, common ground, and similar information. She was less enthusiastic, but she finally agreed. Great—I finally had the shrink of my dreams, and she could now help me deal with the very annoying man who came with the deal.

Here was a different kind of triangle—not sexual, per se—but more insidious. All my conversations with the Boyfriend were about our different, and occasionally mutual, therapy. In bed with Mom we certainly were—trouble was, I came to love Mom more than I loved him, while he remained convinced that he was her most cherished client. Just like when a man has bought three lap dances from a stripper, has a raging hard-on, and declares in all seriousness, "I think she really likes me!"

When I initiated mistressing, our dear therapist announced that one of us had to go—or both. If we were potentially not monogamous and she knew it, the therapy would be poisoned. The Boyfriend announced that he'd had enough therapy and was ready to hit the road alone, comforted by the notion that when a man chooses his lover over his therapist it is a sign of his newly found independence and maturity. This was fortunate because I announced that I would definitely not give up the shrink no matter what. I chose my therapist over my lover, which was a sign of my own growing maturity: I had finally decided to choose a woman over a man.

After four or five months of mistressing, I ended it completely and during the last phone call with the Boyfriend the elegant irony became apparent: he had now lost not only his lover but his shrink as well.

I see it like this: you just never really can know what a particular connection is about—until later. The Last Boyfriend was about me finding a woman who would not only witness and analyze my misery but whose very presence in my life echoed my never-before-possible ability to endorse myself above, and beyond, any man. And when A-Man entered my world, she endorsed me from behind as well—while I learned to embrace my masochism sexually and leave it out of my life.

DURING

A-MAN

You just don't know when he's going to show up. The one who is going to change everything forever, the one who's going to rock your world. He might even be someone you already know.

The Young Man had been gone for two years. In the meantime, I had acquired the Boyfriend, while the redhead Pre-Raphaelite had acquired a tall, skinny, rocker musician who wore more makeup than she did: they painted each other's nails and were mad in monogamous love. So when the Young Man called, I knew it would have to be a two-way; the safety of a three-way sandwich was no longer an option.

I was petrified. My male dilemma was personified in these two men before me: the Boyfriend was dependable in life but not in sex, while the Young Man was dependable in sex but not in life. Can't a woman win? My experiments so far said no. The Boyfriend was too safe, too arrogant, too possessive. But the Young Man was too dangerous, too sexy, too young, too not here. But I had Rule #3 at my disposal, so at least he was legal, technically.

In fact, the decision to see the Young Man the very afternoon he called was surprisingly easy. Earlier that day, the Boyfriend had juiced up my anger to the point of murderous rage by pontificating about "our" relationship—he was in "our" relationship alone, as far as I was concerned. And so it was arranged. It was three, the Young Man would be over at four. Love in the afternoon, like Gary Cooper and Audrey Hepburn. Well, not quite. I didn't have a cello.

With one hour to prepare, I had no time to think. Just as well, because there was no sense in it. But the ones who made sense drove me crazy. I had already caught several men desiring matrimony—and married the best of them—and had found misery to spare. Catching a man and hauling him to the altar was not what I wanted. I had a creepy suspicion that all those "proposals" were more about insecurities and jealousies than about love, more about tying me down emotionally when I needed tying down physically. I didn't want a lifetime commitment; I wanted a sexual commitment. For a few hours, anyway.

Trembling, I got on my knees, not knowing what else to do, and prayed to my unknown God to allow me to surrender to this man, in this moment, for this afternoon only. No more. I could not imagine more. I can only fuck one fuck at a time. Could I have the courage to not be afraid of the beauty of the Young Man just this once? To go all the way in with him, not knowing if there was a way out? I got up off my knees and turned on the bath.

I bathed, shaved my legs, powdered my whole body with honey dust, set up the music, closed the curtains, fed the cat, lit the incense and candles, and then—very excited, very apprehensive—I put myself into a black thong, a black bra, and a long black velvet gown.

∞

The doorbell rang, late. I opened the door and he stepped inside and then stepped inside of me. He folded me into his big arms, no words, and pressed me close. I was his from that moment forth. I allowed it, and then it took on a life of its own. For the next three hours, I melted into this man in a way I never had with any man before.

As his cock entered me to the full, the pressure made me flinch. He looked down at me and said gently, "I won't hurt you." Actually, it did hurt—he had a big cock—but somehow I understood intuitively that it wasn't *about* hurting me, it was about something else. As with dancing, I knew that I had to work with my discomfort, embrace it, to get to the next level.

And then he fucked me in the ass. Is this what he learned while out of town? It was the first time for me. Ever. My God, he was good. I mean bad. What nerve he had. So graceful. It was very slow, very careful, very connected and painful. It was here, in there, that I first tasted the experience of moving through pain and fear to that plateau on the other side where I met this man in a foreign land called Bliss. Bliss is not a pain-free zone; it is a postpain zone. Big difference.

His cock inside me on that virgin voyage was an emotional and anatomical miracle: the impossible had come to pass in my ass. Now God had my total attention. If I had walked on water I couldn't have been more amazed. This was my first act of sacrifice that was not mired in the vicious circle of self-reflective narcissism, the first that delivered me to an entirely new place, instead of a new angle on the old one. I have been changed ever since. Forever changed. And it began physically with his cock in my ass—the act that proposed the mystery—and psychically with my decision to allow it, the best one I ever made. I simply wanted to let this particular man into me, literally. I wanted who he was deep inside who I was.

Of course, it also took his balls, the balls to want and try and dare to fuck me in my tiny, tight ass. I'll respect him forever for that. Finally, a man who was not afraid. The Young Man, 3-Way Man, was transfigured before my eyes. A-Man was born.

Something else happened that first afternoon. I stopped mourning my marriage. The mourning ceased, I believe, because someone else had entered my consciousness deeply enough to override the grief, transforming the previous loss into a blessing, making space for a new entry. No one had tried my back door before. That was where my power resided and where it shifted. As hostess at my front door, I was, as you now know, the critical Queen, the impossible Princess, the angry child. But with A-Man in my ass, I became sweet again. So sweet.

Within days, I told the Boyfriend that we were done. All done. I couldn't be sweet with him, only mad. He may have resided in "reality," but those three hours with A-Man clarified everything for me: "reality" was not my home.

WHY THERE?

Once gravity reasserted its hold on me, I immediately started examining my experience. It felt like my new job. I'd been given a gift and now I had to attempt some understanding. Why? Why me? Why him? Why *there?*

I had given my vaginal virginity to the first man who paid me any consistent sexual attention. I would have married him as only a virgin would: with adoration and ignorance. Eight penises later, I married one. Ten years later, when I departed that union, I was horny as hell, like never before—a bunny on a hot tin roof—but intercourse was not what I wanted. I needed love, admiration, and pussy worship. This insatiable desire ruled my life. But then A-Man came along and shook my overanalyzed ego off its self-important pedestal.

I was an anal virgin. He showed me, physically, where my rage resided. Anger thrives in your ass. A Dickensian alley, the ass. Despite its tiny, ignored entry, once opened, it contains literally yard upon yard of coiled past traumas, the internal gripping of the emotionally unbearable. A-Man penetrated the site of my anger and cauterized my wound.

I was now being given a second chance—not on the well-trodden vaginal trail, but in a place entirely new to my consciousness—and it quickly became the site of my consciousness. Truly virgin, once again. With the discovery of this new world, I experienced all the wonder and beauty that a deflowering might be but rarely is.

And so it began, in naive complicity, once a week, twice a week, three times a week. Mostly late afternoons. He was an expert and I was willing. I began to count. It just seemed like the right thing to do.

#41

Ablaze afterward, he stood up, still hard, and slugged some water from a blue bottle.

"What is it about?" I asked from the bed, flushed and dazed.

He stopped drinking, looked over at me, paused, and said, "Vibrations."

He says we're learning something about time. The passage of time, the experience of time, the truth of time, the eternity of time. The best time.

ENTERING THE EXIT

Once initiated, I couldn't help thinking about anal everything. Including the mechanics. The digestive system is a one-way pipe where peristaltic contractions urge food from mouth to anus. Assfucking entails the bold—and contrary—attempt to travel the route in reverse.

Fucking a pussy is entering a cave with only one pinprick exit—the hole in the cervix that enters the womb. (And, of course, it is an "exit" to parenthood.) Under normal circumstances, the pussy is a pretty closed, if expandable, place. The vagina is a receptacle. The anal canal, on the other hand, is directly, though complexly, connected to the mouth, the point of entry, the place that feeds the life. Thirty feet or so of digestive track from rectum to colon to small intestine to stomach to esophagus to throat to mouth is the route entered by the anal fucker.

A-Man and I exist in the land beyond the intercourse that breeds babies. That is good, too, don't get me wrong. We do that, too, warm-up. But we live in the land beyond, behind. The place where depth is infinite and the love seems infinite, ever growing. Deep penetration, deep love. The physical depth somehow leads into that other depth as if my soul slept in my bowels and is now awakened.

The directions are clear: if you want to procreate enter the front door, but if you really want to become a part of a woman's internal workings, to penetrate her being most deeply, the back door is your portal. Anxiety, that ever-present agony, exists because of the inescapable knowledge that all must end. Enter an ass and you enter a passage that does not end. It is the exit to infinity. The back door to liberty.

Besides, pussies have just been through too much. Give them a rest. They are old news—tired, betrayed, overused, reused, abused—and have been overly publicized, politicized, and redeemed. They are no longer naughty, no longer the place for defiance, rebellion, or rebirth. Pussies are now too politically correct. The ass is where it's at: the playground for anarchists, iconoclasts, artists, explorers, little boys, horny men, and women desperate to relinquish, even temporarily, the power that has been so hard won and cruelly awarded by the feminist movement. Ass-fucking realigns the balance for a woman with too much power—and a man with too little. (I think this explains the prevalence of butt-fucking in heterosexual porn: masses of men, refugees from feminism, watching, hard and ever-hopeful.)

In his forays inside me, A-Man hits new walls, new angles, new ends, and that self-preserving voice of "too much" echoes through my brain as I feel a kind of pressure, a resistance. But I have never said "too much." Never. I breathe through, adjust the angle, and stay where he pushes until I open and receive him in farther. I expand into him and the pain subsides, transforms, into a profound sensation of freedom—freedom from pain, freedom to be crazy, freedom to harmonize with the universe. This is all physical. And it is the birth of love. His cock is my laser healer. Every point it probes inside me pierces my armor, the armor of self-protection, and the two fears—love and death—momentarily lose their grip and I experience a moment of immortality.

#75

Vertical fucking. Upside down, legs over my head, knees by my ears, ass up, he perches over me like an acrobat and points his cock down into me. He thrusts downward to Earth's center, and I am grounded. I point upward, outward to the sky, to the Milky Way, to heaven's gate, and I see clearly between my legs his cock pumping like a piston. Angle is everything.

We achieve a kind of gravity-free coordination, complete transcendence of the "fight"—the fight that is life—total trust allowing his deep, hard, long, and fast plunges entirely without self-protective gripping. Undulating . . . and great inner peace as I am rocked like a mermaid in the ocean.

THE DOUBLE-SPHINCTER THEORY

More mechanics: the inner anal sphincter is not within conscious control. It is regulated by the brain in the gut, the enteric nervous system, and is reflexive, opening on demand. The external sphincter, the internal's sister sphincter, is, however, connected to the conscious brain, regulated by conscious control—witness the ability to grip and hold when necessary, when angry, when scared, when stressed. Unconscious internal sphincter, conscious external sphincter, only centimeters apart. Where else is one's unconscious and conscious mind so intimately connected, so readily regulated, so easily probed? It is a psychological playground of the most intriguing potential. Put an ass on the couch and much is revealed.

But the external sphincter did not begin with consciousness. For the first year or so of life it was unconscious, reacting in conjunction with the internal and letting go on demand—hence diapers. The brain and spinal cord at birth are not yet developed enough for conscious control.

And then comes toilet training. When the brain is sophisticated enough and the parents encourage (or scream) enough, the little eighteen-month-old becomes conscious of that external anal sphincter and learns to grip it, control it, and not to let the shit fly at every urge. Shame is born. All this is to say that when I get fucked in the ass, I have learned to play with, and even reverse, that long-ago, probably traumatic coming to consciousness about gripping my ass, holding on to it, showing it to no one. After all, Freud hypothesized that one's shit is the first gift one offers one's parents—one's first creative production.

Only now—ninety-seven ass fucks later—is the enormity of the power that lies in this area dawning on me. It is emotional and physical therapy on the deepest level: revisiting and literally learning to trust enough to open the forbidden exit and enter the forbidden zone. As a baby, the first big resounding NO from the world as we know it is the NO perpetrated upon a loose and unconscious external anal sphincter. Getting ass-fucked is the most extreme form of rebellion against one's parents in which one could possibly indulge—returning not to adolescent transgressions, but rather to the original injury.

I experience a regression to a very young age when he's in my ass. I goo and gaa and giggle and feel the joy that must have existed before anxiety took over. As if all I ever wanted was to be loved while not gripping my ass, but allowing it to be as it is. And what is released along with my anal sphincter? A love that is enormous, a love waiting decades to be released, a love that flows freely, a love that is infinite at the moment of its conception.

Okay, I understand. You're thinking: Infinite love is good, but what if I bleed en route? To be on the safe side I have never not used a condom, but I have also never, ever bled. This can be a question of the skill of one's lover but it also may be that some assholes, like mine, are just more able, more resilient, than others—a genetic blessing. If you bleed, don't do it. I wouldn't. Period.

I also know that when some of you hear anal sex you see nothing but shit—shit, shit everywhere. Shit on the bed, shit on his cock, shit on your ass. I am here to tell you it just isn't like that. Hardly a trace, ever. All you have to do is include in your regular bathing a nice little finger-in-the-ass bath prior to an anal visitation. What woman doesn't wash her pussy before sex? Same thing, just rinse out your ass, too. Shit is not my thing, either—don't want to see it, smell it, or clean it up. Ass-fucking is not about shit. It's about not being afraid of your shit, going past your shit—to find the shit that matters.

#98

*He fucked me in the ass at 11:20 last night so long, so hard, so
smooth, so hilariously, so slowly, so fast, so very, very deep. After
forty-five minutes of this he says, "Now I'm gonna fuck your pussy."
And he fucked my pussy 360 degrees around. Then he says, "I'm
gonna get me some sacred spot." And he does, anointing my sacred
place—the grave of my past—with his blasphemous baptismal
juice.*

"I think it's your greatest gift," he says after.

"What is?"

"Submission."

PROFILE OF AN ASS-FUCKER

Ass-fucking a woman is clearly about authority. The man's authority; the woman's complete acceptance of it. A man must have this confidence, in himself and his cock, to fuck a woman in the ass. If he does not have this control, his cock will direct the action; he will move too quickly, hurt the once-willing woman, and rarely, rightly, will he be given a second chance.

Why A-Man has this authority I do not know. Psychology might find childhood reasons, but I believe, ultimately, that it's something God-given, a deep knowledge of personal responsibility. This kind of self-possession and lack of desperation can get a man a long way with a woman . . . or at least partway up her ass. In the end, it's who you are that will get you somewhere. Or nowhere.

He told me once that he likes being where he shouldn't be, crossing the velvet rope, hand in the candy jar, late to work, cock in my ass, an ass too small for his cock. A-Man made it so deeply into my ass because he dared. No one else really tried. Anyone who dares to be that intimate, that crazy, well, he might just get somewhere he never got before.

I am in the throes of coming at the moment of first touch, my body, pussy, ass so open they peel outwardly to suck him in. I was never that open before. If I were that open to someone else, would I feel the same joy of openness? No. They would annoy me long before I was that open. It's all that yakking that ruins it; it reveals too much. A-Man is the least annoying man I've ever known. And the only one who never yields to my will.

At the same time, contrary to easy supposition, I do not believe that it is the arrogant, macho man who is the great ass-fucker: he is the asshole. That guy probably doesn't even like women, he's too busy competing with other men. In my limited experience, the great ass-fucker is the patient, gentle man, the one who knows how to listen to a woman, how to be with a woman, and has the equipment that can slow her down. He is the one who can imaginatively experience her submission—her release of control—with her, and thus know precisely how to get her to that place: he absorbs all that she gives up. He is a kind man, A-Man.

OBITUARY

After such a stunning start, I prepared, as any bright woman would, for the end. Great love always brings thoughts of death and separation. This was a war—between decency and desire, between convention and pleasure, between me, myself, and I—and that great aphrodisiac fueled my craving. With the assumption, or expectation, of longevity gone, the moat of self-protection and the apathy of safety disappear and passion floods the world. Well, it flooded mine, anyway. Now is all there was, all I had—and I knew it.

The aphoristic obituary was especially comforting. My testimony would serve if he died, if I died, or—worst of all—if he flaked on me.

> He had the biggest, hardest, and most gentle cock I ever knew.
> He was the one who fucked me in the ass, missionary-style, before he fucked my pussy.
> He was the one who looked beautiful to me when we fucked, the others all looked like men with contorted faces—best not to look.
> He didn't grunt, or groan, or squeak during sex. He beamed

and glowed, eyes wide open, shaking his head, saying, "Wow! Wow!" and then he'd fuck me some more.

He was the thirty-third man, and the only one I really liked to fuck. The others were just men and I allowed it. Resentfully.

Most men fuck in and out, in and out, in and out, on and on. But he fucked like he was actually going somewhere. And he was.

He was the only one who took time to be friends with my cat. The others regarded my little fur ball as a hindrance, an obstacle, even a threat. They just didn't get it: love me, love my pussy.

He was my blood.

He was the one who never got real.

He was the one I never conquered.

He was one I had the most fun with.

He had the only cock I worshiped.

He was the one with whom I couldn't tell whose pleasure gave me more pleasure. With the others my pleasure was the only pleasure.

He was the guy who could fuck for three hours . . . and still not come.

He was the one who showed me real physical joy. The others just made me come. With him I came to . . . the Kingdom.

He was sweet-sweet-sweet.

He was the one who oozed love. Through his fingertips, his movement, his skin, and his cock.

He gave me nothing outside of bed. In bed he gave me everything that I, as a woman, could ever desire.

He fucked like a rolling ocean.

I didn't have those powerful but so brief and geographically specific outward climaxes with him, it was the building of an inward tidal wave that flooded my body, my brain, and then spilled into my soul.

He never, unlike the others, asked me to be "his"—but I was.

He was the one who treated me like his—in bed. All the others treated me like theirs out of bed, but in bed I could smell their fear.

With him sex was about transcendence, with the others power.

He swooped in and out of my pussy, my ass, my life. Others smothered, wishing, foolishly, to colonize what they coveted.

Fucking him was like breathing in wide open space.

If I never loved again I would die having known a big, big love.

There was always that moment when he fucked me when all my thoughts ceased and turned to God: I was entering His territory.

He didn't please me. He possessed me.

He, you see, was the one I really loved.

Having now imagined its demise, I mustered the courage to proceed with the affair.

#101

He stands by the bed naked, hard, and beautiful and says, "Show me your pussy." He watches as I take off my thong, lie back on the bed, and bend my knees up and apart. Looking at my pussy, he says, "Spread it apart." With a hand on each side I open my little pink pussy lips to him. He kneels before me and sucks on my clit, sings on my clit like a troubadour breaking all the rules. I flowed into his tongue and he murmured, "You like it when I eat your pussy, don't you?"

"I would die for it," I admitted.

I cannot imagine feeling greater love in all my life, nor do I expect to ever feel greater love, except for him. Nor would I ever ask or want greater love than I feel for him.

With any others, after him, I will need to rest.

THE UNWRITTEN RULES

We are not domestic. We stay in the desire, in the bedroom—and out of the kitchen, the laundry, the office, and any other room that would threaten to bring in reality. We have, on a few occasions, when famished after sex, cooked dinner—well, actually he cooked it, but then we ate it in the bathtub with candles, floating a large metal bowl filled with tender rare meat between us. Both of us in the deep end, of course. We've never been to a movie and don't plan on going to one, ever. Why would we? We are the movie: the porn that can never be—visually astounding, spontaneously inventive, genitally graphic, and viscerally soul-searing. It isn't predictable with A-Man. The sex, the ass-fucking, that is the only constant. We never don't fuck.

We are not monogamous. Never have been and never will be. Neither of us has ever asked for it and neither of us has ever offered it. Offering it is the only way it could happen—neither of us would intrude on the other's free choice. Free choice is at the core of what is hot between us. The subject has been discussed only to establish what is mutually understood. "Don't ask, don't tell" is the basic policy. He says, "I don't need to know." He pays attention to what is, not what isn't.

Having never done this before, I thought about it plenty. If one has sex with someone other than the Beloved, what happens? Does one risk diminishing one's affection for the Beloved? Does it contaminate the love? Or does it merely confirm the love in every way, the contrast illuminating the beauty of the Beloved yet again, in yet another way, from yet another angle. And this gift to each other— the freedom to allow for other experiences—only enhances the love. Love without chains is love.

The experience of being truly free, without recrimination, without judgment, to choose at any time, on any day, this one or that one, only reinforces love of the Beloved, reinforces the choice of the Beloved as the Beloved. Not being monogamous, and exercising that option, secures the great love—always being tested, it is confirmed, strengthened, reshaped, redefined.

If a man can possess a woman sexually—really possess—he won't need to control her ideas, her opinions, her clothes, her friends, even her other lovers. In my experience of many lovers, only he has truly possessed me and so set me free. He fucks my ass for hours with a dick an inch too big for the job: *that* is possession. After a round like that he doesn't need to infiltrate my life, my psyche, my time, or my wardrobe, because he has infiltrated the core of my being—the rest is just peripheral decoration. Domination— total and complete domination of my being—that is where I find freedom.

∽

I assumed from the beginning of our affair that he was probably fucking this other woman here or there or somewhere. And he knew that I knew. This was not the Pre-Raphaelite redhead but a pretty, quiet brunette who also exercised at the gym. I was even turned on by the power I assumed he had over her. I knew about her, but she didn't know about me, and this worked just fine. I even had my own fantasies about her. About seducing her myself, about him telling her to eat my pussy while he watched. I ran into her on occasion at the gym and we were always friendly; she seemed like a nice woman, self-effacing.

He and I had even discussed the idea of a three-way with her—we always reminisced fondly about the magic of our times with the red-head and wondered if it could be reproduced with someone else. But he said he was not sure that I would like her body. Proportion is important to me in matters of beauty, and though she was slim, she had no tits and a wide ass. Good enough for him, obviously, but perhaps not for me. A curious assessment, but probably correct.

As time went on, however, this woman became increasingly abstract. A-Man was fucking me so often and so well that she was easily dismissed, often forgotten. That he is free to fuck whomever he likes and yet repeatedly calls me, comes to me, fucks me, seems a greater proof of love and desire on a daily basis than a commitment of monogamy would be—especially if it was made only to prevent insecurities from rising to the surface.

Is his love as deep as mine? I don't care if it is as superficial as mine is deep as long as he, and his rock-hard desire, show up at my back door several times a week. Sodomy ignites a gratitude of great scope. I suspect that until he shattered the control panel of my being—my mental acuity and my physical power—I had never really loved before.

How do you know it's love, real love?

When you meet the one with whom you are not afraid to die. The one who takes away that constant gnawing fear of death and gives one air to breathe.

Not afraid to die, this is the feeling he generates when he fucks my ass. Pussy penetration does not delve this far into my psyche; does not break the barrier; does not stop the fear.

Did the love or the sodomy come first? Love grows from lust. This I know. Besides, I don't trust love. I've heard it declared too often. But I trust lust completely.

#121

After, I say, "Maybe it's not even sex. Something else. Beyond sex."
Did I have a regular battle-to-the-end clitoral orgasm? No. Had I
even thought about it? No. Only a fool would hold on to what she
knows while being shown some land of release beyond orgasm. The
land of harmony, of deep harmony with another human being.
Family. He is my family.

K-Y

"What's your afternoon like?" It begins.

He has an appointment at six, will be over at three. It is now two. One hour. The courtesan takes over. I turn on the bath, all hot, and let it fill.

I check the condom stash and refill it, always having plenty, at least five, more is better, a feeling of bounty, of possibility, like popcorn. I check the K-Y tubes, pushing the insides to the opening end and then rinsing them off under the tap, sticky from last time. The heat rises as I wash those tubes. I use my pink nail brush to wash just under the ridge on the cap where his thumb pushes it open. Dirt always collects there; it's how I know that tube was used. I adore washing those tubes smooth.

In the beginning, I bought the tiny little travel tubes, good for one or two sessions, small, discreet, deniable. Once I knew, initially, the ecstasy of the act, I also knew it could only be a very rare occurrence, sort of like a birthday special. I reasoned that it would not be healthy for my little asshole to be so invaded too frequently. I reasoned that bliss was not free, not plannable, and definitely not something that might come my way very often. Such reasoning led me to buy those little travel tubes. But those tiny tubes kept running out and denial became an effort. Ass-fucking was part of the regular repertoire. The next time he opened the drawer, he pulled out a giant, phallic-sized white-and-blue tube, looked at it, and fell off the bed howling with laughter. It was a risky move for me. Presumptuous. Practical.

After several months of using one large tube after another, I put two large tubes in the drawer at the same time. That is how he developed the ritual of dispersing the tubes while I sucked his cock. The beautiful man with a fierce erection tossing large white-and-blue plastic tubes around the room (wherever we land he can fuck my ass, right there, right then, no reaching): it is an image of promise as close to a guarantee as I've ever known with a man. The gold band on my left ring finger guaranteed far less. Soon there are as many as five tubes in the drawer at one time, each in a different stage of emptiness, the emptier the better.

I still haven't figured out how many ass-fucks per four-ounce tube. Probably about eleven. At $4.19 a tube, that is about 38 cents a fuck . . . add that to the price of a condom (thirty-six for $14.99) at 42 cents, and the best thing in the world costs less than a buck. Then I found the tubes discounted at Costco, two for $4.00, and bought six. That brings the whole affair down to 60 cents per cum shot. (Ass-fuckers: use dark glasses for K-Y shopping and don't turn around in the checkout line: they're all staring at your butt in disbelief.)

I'm going to buy stock in K-Y. The Lexus of lubricants. Grateful for the smooth ride.

I heard a television talk-show shrink quizzing a cross-dressing man to test if he was gay or straight. Playing quick word association, she says "football," he says "beer"; she says . . . he says . . . she says "KY," he says "Kentucky." She announces triumphantly that he is heterosexual. And, I would add, clearly not a heterosexual sodomite.

Of the liquid lubricants, Astroglide is king. But be forewarned: if you pour Astroglide onto K-Y during a single vigorous ass-fucking, then expect a large amount of froth. Froth everywhere.

What do the K and Y stand for? According to Johnson & Johnson, which has been manufacturing the jelly since 1910—their service reps were very friendly on the phone—they don't stand for anything, just arbitrary letters assigned by the original research scientists. But they have come to mean plenty.

TRACELESS

Now that I have fallen into both sin and love, my scribbled daily testimonies serve to keep my anxiety of loss just barely at bay. With him I live on the ledge of the abyss. The terror that this experience might end competes with the even worse terror that it might be lost forever.

Because he and I are not fused, except during sexual contact, I must constantly confront the spaces between us. He never overstays his welcome, and thus cultivates an air of scarcity, an erotic component of powerful and paradoxical consequences. On the one hand, the element of instability is clearly an essential factor, perhaps the central factor, in generating the total thrill of each and every encounter. The lost heat that monogamous couples constantly mourn is always there for us. And yet this unpredictability also leaves me with ample time and space for the insecurities of love to blossom. Thus I doubt, I question, I worry and heap indignities upon myself for which there is neither evidence nor refutation. The lingering voice of convention is always attempting to diminish and deride my own transcendent experience. And yet I have never tried to control him in order to avoid this anxiety; I have always known that he is not an extension of me but a clearly separate human being.

Besides, I am well aware by now that if a man exhibits too many signs of attachment I lose interest and the sex becomes laden with obligation. Desire is sexy, a show of free will; attachment is the enemy of free will. A-Man, with his scarcity, has become the first man to keep me poised at that delectable point where I both thrive and suffer: always-in-desire, never-having-enough.

It is easier to want something than to have it—and so often when you do get the thing you've wanted so long, you're busy with numerous substitutes. With him somehow the wanting and the having combine, simultaneously. He is my very real yet eternally impossible fantasy: a man I can respect.

Living entirely in the moment, he leaves no traces. He is here when he is here. He is gone when he is gone. Others linger when they are gone, like a bad smell, even when they were never really here in the first place. He is the most present, and as a result, the most emphatically, painfully absent.

He recoils from nostalgia, detects sentimentality across a room, and the only hard evidence of our encounters is his relentlessly hard cock. Hardly something a girl can hang on to after the act. He keeps his private life private. I've not met his friends and do not know what he does during time not spent with me. He rejects gossip, refuses photographs, and eschews the love note. He is not a romantic, he is a practitioner of the here and now. He acts like a man unafraid of death—or else joyously defiant. I, however, am mortified by my mortality, and so I scribble on and on, searching for evidence, creating evidence, of our affair.

He says he doesn't need devotion. He says he doesn't even really need to be listened to. If he isn't heard the first time, he'll say it again. What he does want, he says, is the adventure, the ride together, the opportunity to enter a time warp with someone.

A-Man is a man with many tools. He can hang a mirror with toggle bolts, clean a skylight, grill a rack of lamb, pose naked in the garden like a Rodin sculpture, and fuck my ass. He's a doer, not a thinker, and he openly admits that he wants a woman to be smarter than he is. I have never before met a guy brave enough to want that. It is the confidence of a man who owns his cock and knows exactly what to do with it and where to put it. Thinkers, in my experience, can't fuck; they're too busy with the meaning and the metaphors, too busy avoiding their tool, afraid of entering a hole without a clearly marked exit. He is an underthinker—and overfucker. A-Man leaves the meaning of the metaphors to me.

He has given me almost no material gifts. Except one. A twelve-pack stack of yellow legal pads. I am writing on one now. Smart guy.

Why him? Four things:

1) He loves me.
2) He knows how to fuck me.
3) He doesn't take me seriously.
4) He is not afraid of me.

No one else had all four. Most only had the first, and even that was usually merely a sentiment, not a course of action. If you love me you shall fuck me without fear. I don't want to be a whore to a man's insecurities. I want to be a whore to my own.

STATISTICS

Enough—for now—of my story. What about yours? I am not alone, you know, in my sometimes unlawful obsession. Despite the landmark 2003 Supreme Court decision *Lawrence v. Texas* that renders all antisodomy laws unconstitutional and unenforceable, the statutes are still on the books in twenty-two states and Puerto Rico (and I suspect that Disneyland has an ordinance somewhere in the fine print). Every state in the Union had an antisodomy law until 1962, when Illinois became the first state to repeal the law. A steady spread of repeals in twenty-seven more states and the District of Columbia followed—good to know that all that ass-fucking in the nation's capital has finally been legalized.

Of the states where antisodomy laws can still be found in the legal literature, Kansas, Missouri, Oklahoma, and Texas are unique in that "the unspeakable vice of the Greeks" remains illegal only for homosexuals, whereas Alabama, Florida, Idaho, Louisiana, Michigan, Mississippi, North Carolina, South Carolina, Utah, and Virginia forbid it no matter what your sex—or species.

Definitions vary: in Rhode Island, for example, where the law was repealed in 1998, sodomy was a felony, an "abominable and detestable crime against nature" meriting seven to twenty years in jail—unless, of course, you were married. Then it was totally okay. To think that you had to get married to get legally "abominable and detestable." I really respect that sort of legal logic.

South Carolina is the only state that still defines sodomy as "buggery," an affectionate nod, I assume, to the state's original position as a British colony. This state also claims the impressive distinction of the most prosecutions: between 1954 and 1974, there were no less than 146 buggery cases, resulting in 125 convictions.

A 1977 attempt in Oklahoma to repeal its antisodomy law was unsuccessful due to a vote-delaying "chorus of giggles," according to the official records. In Arkansas, where sodomy was defined as a misdemeanor only for homosexuals, the bill was explicitly "aimed at weirdos and queers who live in a fairyland world and are trying to wreck family life." Good thing this law was declared unconstitutional in 2002, if only to deflect attention from the Arkansas legislature's propensity for queer and weirdo prose.

Minnesota gets high marks for animal rights: there was once a curious addendum to their law, since repealed, stating that sex "between humans and birds" is strictly prohibited—sounds like some sick fuck got his chicks confused. As a woman who prefers most animals to most people, I will say without reservation that I think this particular statute should be reinstated to prosecute those particular Homo sapiens who threaten the avian community.

The penalties that accompanied these laws varied widely: in

Utah, you could get off with a penalty of a thousand dollars, rendering the state one of the cheaper places in the Union in which to perform illegal sodomy. Back in 1857, a twenty-one-year-old Mormon man was ordered shot to death for "bestiality" with his horse, but, in a brutal reversal, the Mormon was spared while the horse was shot. Very sensible.

Speaking of Utah, I can't help wondering how Mormons feel about anal sex—with humans, that is—what with all those extra wives and orifices around the house. Does one prohibited penchant for multiple options lead to another?

One had to be very careful, however, in adjacent Idaho, where the same act could get you life in the slammer with all the other newly converted sodomites. This huge variable of penalty in such close geographic proximity suggests that the hundred-and-fifty-mile border between Utah and Idaho might be packed with cheap motels—Buggery Row—filled with Idahoans enjoying some bargain borderline behavior.

Despite its new legal status, sodomy remains the last taboo, sexually and socially. Oprah Winfrey talks about everything—rape, child molestation, incest, adultery, murder, drugs, homosexuality, bisexuality, even threesomes—but never, ever, about sodomy except in the guise of abuse and criminal behavior. Always a scandal, never an advertisement. "Odd how nineteeth-century literature is sealed off at both ends by an anal scandal," the theater critic Kenneth Tynan observed. "Wilde up Bosie's bum, Byron up Annabella's."

All this evidence leads me to believe that entering the exit will never become mainstream. Even the spell-checker on my computer that recognizes more than 135,000 words does not recognize *sodomize*. But that's okay. I know how to spell it.

PUBLIC INTEREST

There is, however, a growing underground movement of heterosexual backdoor behavior, according to the largest and most authoritative national survey of sexual behavior ever published in the United States. "Our data shows that anal sex was much more prevalent than might have been expected," begins the dry admission from the unsuspecting researchers. Overall, 25 percent of men and women try it in their lifetimes, and 10 percent have done so in the last year. Only 2 percent, however, on their "most recent" encounter—I just love statistics.

Nevertheless, between the ages of thirty and fifty, the likelihood of male heterosexual sodomy rises to a respectable one third of all men. One out of three. Think about it next time you're at a party and looking around the room. A curious footnote points out that all these percentages are only based on men's and women's two primary sex partners. Meaning: if someone is having anal sex with their #3 lover, then it is not reflected in these figures. Does it not count as statistically valid behavior if you're anal only with #3? Why are they not included? I suspect foul play. Who paid for this survey anyway? Or, perhaps, the trackers were onto a hidden truth: whoever is fucking your ass is never gonna be #3 or even #2. Ass-fuckers are always #1.

When they start breaking down the anal prospectors into socio-economic categories, things get even more interesting. The higher the level of education, the more anal sex. What are they teaching in college these days?

Unsurprisingly perhaps, both male and female atheists are the most likely backdoor enthusiasts, but the Catholics run a very close second. For the former it is pleasure, perversion, and possibly their only chance for the religious experience of submission; for the latter, no doubt, it's merely birth control.

While white women are the most common sodomitic recipients (Sue Johanson, Canada's Dr. Ruth, says 43 percent of all women have tried anal sex), their male counterparts appear not to be their most likely perpetrator. Hispanic men are the white woman's most likely ride for a trip to the other side. To think that anal sex actually encourages integration!

Perhaps even more politically correct is the less mainstream, but nevertheless significant, "bend-over boyfriend" movement. This movement certainly deserves . . . ah . . . well, these guys must deserve something for facing not only the terror of homosexuality but a girlfriend wielding a dildo bigger than their own dicks. And what a movement it is! The chance to be a girl, the chance to find out just how much submission it takes to have a hard, seven-inch cock up your bum. Come on, guys, bend over . . . take it like a man.

And there it is: the curious double standard common to so many straight men: terrified of getting it, but all too eager to give it. What is that about? How can they expect a woman to take a cock up her ass when they squeal if anything larger than a pinky finger is waved in their direction? Not that I'd want any man of mine to be bending over too eagerly. Definitely not. Protest is the only dignified position for a straight man to assume when he's consented to be ass-fucked. Protest every inch of the way, I say.

There is plenty of protest in Eve Ensler's popular play *The Vagina Monologues*. But why is it that in all those interviews, all those questions, all those monologues, there is not a single mention of a woman's asshole? So close and yet so far; the space that could change the world. All that "liberated" Pussy Talk, and yet so avoidant about what lies behind their sacred place: the hole of no return. Oh, well. It would be treason, I suppose, to advocate surrender at the rear for those who are just finally claiming victory at the front. Victory from behind, however, seems so much more, how can I put it . . . honorable. I can't but wonder if my play, *The Anal Dialogues*, could find a venue even off-off-off-Broadway? Perhaps in some dark performance space down some little-traveled back alley?

Clearly, yelling about butt-fucking from the rooftops—or on the national radio waves—is not advised. In April 2004, it was proposed that Clear Channel Communications, the nation's largest radio broadcaster, be fined no less than $495,000 by the Federal Communications Commission for a single twenty-minute segment of the *Howard Stern Show* in which Stern discussed, at some length, what he refers to as "anal." (It probably didn't help matters that the conversation was frequently punctuated by fart noises.) Thank God that having anal sex is so much cheaper than talking about it.

Despite this new trend of sodomitic censorship, ass-fucking has made several auspicious appearances recently on screens both big and small. The subject came up regularly in the popular TV series *Sex and the City*, whose heroines discussed not only men's growing interest in "the ass" but also their own willingness to accommodate those interests, the appropriateness of doing so on a first date, and the basic lube how-tos. Perhaps even more surprising was its mention in the Hollywood hit *Bridget Jones's Diary*. At one point, when Bridget is lying in bed after having sex with her caddish lover, Daniel Cleaver, she reminds him that what they just did is illegal in several countries. To which he replies, without missing a beat, that that's one of the reasons he's so pleased to be living in England today.

Is Daniel Cleaver the latest incarnation of the bad-boy lover, the zipless fuck for the twenty-first century? After all, the zipless ass-fuck simply takes zipless to a new hole level. So does missionary-position ass-fucking. The term itself conjures up such perfect contradiction: the most patriarchal position, the most biblically sanctioned, and yet, well, what a difference an inch can make. The experience on the other hand—best achieved with a nice firm pillow under the ass—makes me feel downright missionary. After all, here I am spreading the word, sharing the epiphany like a born-again believer, a convert, an anal zealot.

#145 and #146

We just completed both 145 and 146 consecutively in the course of an hour and a half. He never went down. I grabbed the base of his cock shortly after he had pulled out and shot vertically up my arched back, arcing over my face. His jizz landed squarely on a black velvet pillow with a satisfying splat. That look was still in his eye, that crazy fucking look, and I asked, "May I lick your cock?"

"Yes," he said gently, generously. And we did the whole thing all over again. Double bliss, double cum, exponential fun.

GETTING READY

If you want the whole thing, the Gods will give it to you.
But you must be ready for it.

—JOSEPH CAMPBELL

I dry the freshly washed K-Y tubes on my bath towel and put them back in the bedside drawer. I turn off the bathwater and strip into the wet heat. Knees drawn up, I fill my pussy with water and shoot it out like an underwater fountain. I watch the ripples in the water, sometimes lifting my hips so I can watch the fountain above water. After soaking, soaping, and shaving, I pull the plug, crouch on two feet, and with a slightly soaped middle finger reach gently into my ass and give it a good warm water bath. You could eat out of my ass, and on my ass; it's that clean.

Out of the tub I dry, cream, and powder my entire body—calves, thighs, ass, stomach, arms, neck, breasts—brush my teeth and hair, perfume my wrists and neck, and stain my lips red with a liquid rose potion.

I prepare the bedroom, clearing all books, papers, magazines, and remotes off the bed and piling the pillows at one end. From the closet I retrieve Pink Square, a rectangular pillow I bought because I liked its fleur-de-lis pattern. It doesn't match the colors of the other pillows, but it fits perfectly under my hips, raising them to cock height. It is one of A-Man's favorite amenities and once, when I forgot to put it on the bed, there was a moment when I saw him scanning the bedroom, perturbed: "Where's Pink Square?"

I go in my closet and plan an outfit. Sometimes a black bra and thong, or, occasionally, crotchless panties when I want to be a slut. Applied slutdom doesn't do much for A-Man, though, he just smiles indulgently when he sees those dainty crotchless wonders. But they don't turn him off, either.

A long silk or velvet gown, elegant but easily raised, is the most frequent choice. If I'm feeling like more exposure, I'll choose high, tight shorts and a skimpy top. Lady or slut, I wear high-heeled mules and keep them on throughout—or, at least, I try to. The sound of those shoes hitting the floor, pounded off me, one by one, is his sign that things are going well, that now we're rocking, that now she's lost control of her facade, her fears, even her shoes. It's usually when he's deep in my ass that I can't cling any longer to those heels.

I lay out my outfit on the bed and fill a couple of water bottles and place them around the room and open him a cold beer. I draw the curtains and light candles—at least ten of them. Frankincense adds to the smoke, the chapel is prepared for his confession—and my baptism. I turn off the phone machine and turn on the music. I gravitate to New Age spiritual and chanting monks—to which he comments with a grin, "Oh, we're having a holy fuck today?"—or Leonard Cohen or Tom Waits groaning as only they can: with inimitable angst. But Ella singing Gershwin is best. Ella is sexy but not slight, happy but not saccharine, serious yet funny—and completely subversive. Ella lilts, she taught me how. She is all about floozies, trollops, Delilah, and "boy-and-girl enjoyment." But in the end it's the rhythms. They are blow-job rhythms. Ella inspired me to suck cock like she sings—smooth, easy, deep, surprising, naughty, indulgent, clear.

Then the final cue. The phone rings and he whispers into my ear, "It's Time." This gives me ten minutes for the final ritual. Pussy shaving. I do this last, out of habit. In the beginning I was so distrustful that he would really show up, so unwilling to believe that I could have this pleasure yet again, that until I got that final call I was too fearful to shave. I wouldn't want to coif my mound for nothing. A freshly prepped pussy without a party to attend is a sad site indeed. It would be more disappointment than I could bare. So I shave last.

I am naked now, but in high heels. Can't shave my pussy without the heels on, never have, ever. They elongate my legs, turning my body into an easel displaying the canvas, my crotch, for the upcoming design. It makes me think of Jackson Pollock for some reason—though I am more precise than he in my execution.

Taking two new pink Daisy razors out of the drawer, I remove the plastic protective tip from the first one. I line up the tools: mirror, baby powder, aloe gel.

At this defining moment, ready to commit, but before the first cut, I always read the William Blake poem I keep on the bathroom windowsill in a tiny green-and-gold frame. It is called "Eternity."

He who binds to himself a joy
Does the wingèd life destroy;
But he who kisses the joy as it flies
Lives in eternity's sun rise.

This four-line poem is the reason I have had the courage day after day, month after month, to lay aside my fear of loss and proceed with A-Man in the present, the only place we exist together. In these lines I find the courage to shave my pussy, risking my dignity with every passage of the razor. Each swipe of the blades reveals my vulnerability far more than my sex. I bet Bill Blake never thought his profound little ditty would find such practical use for so profane an act on such sacred ground. Never mind, he is my seer.

Now, pussy trimming is an interesting subject. I am a complete believer. Trim down that wild bush, girls, let him get a view, let him get access. Waxing doesn't really work. It's good for a week, but then there's three weeks of bumps and stubble till you can wax again. I cannot tolerate bumps and stubble for three weeks. So I shave, every single time. I do it dry, using lots of baby powder and two new two-blade disposable razors each time. Against the grain, but gently. It never cuts and never takes off a layer of skin like wet shaving.

Then there's shape. I began with the simple side trims, the tutu trim, from my ballet-dancing days—a nice isosceles triangle. But then I went to a few strip clubs and got jealous of those very exposed, hairless pussies. Now I shave everything in between, smooth, smooth lips, and leave a nice little triangle on top—though carefully, carefully I trim on either side of the top of my slit, just to highlight and expose the magic crevice—very sexy, very porn. On the bed, legs over the head, mirror in hand, I shave the few hairs around my ass—smooth as a baby. I have, with this view, really come to see what he sees, what he loves, where he goes. My rosebud—not Citizen Kane's.

I dress. There are three firm knocks on the door. I'm ready.

New Year's Arithmetic

Eighty-four anal fucks this year—that averages 7 per month, that's 1.75 a week, one every 4.3 days. But he was out of town 21 weeks, in town 31 weeks, which averages 2.7 ass-fucks a week, which makes one every 2.6 days. I like the math; I do it to believe. Me and the Marquis de Sade: he counted, too.

HIS COCK

I always found cocks rather ugly—better not to look too closely. Wrinkled, asymmetrical, disparate shades of color. Dangling and silly when down, curved, veiny, and just plain weird when up. Was this foreign protuberance supposed to get me wet? Visually, it dried me up. Visually, it was humorous. And scary. And they all want you to lick it, suck it, and rub it. Ugh. The only thing I liked about it was the metaphor, a monument of vertical desire. And that unruly hair all over the place. It's insulting. When I deigned to go down on a man, hairs always caught on my tongue—and it can take ages to find that one curly culprit. In short, a cock was not a thing of beauty to me.

Now, women, they are beautiful. Breasts, hips, curves, asses, faces, eyes, lips, smell, pussy—everything about a beautiful woman is, well, beautiful. Would my eyes ever see a cock as an object of beauty? I tolerated them at worst and felt a mild, passing affection at best. And since they rarely did much for me during intercourse, I really had no proper place for them.

Then he came along and it all changed—in those first three

hours. The epiphany of the cock. I love his cock. Every millimeter, every centimeter, every movement at every moment. His was the first that spoke to me, that took me personally, that never failed me. A-Man remains calm in the face of his own erection—the ultimate test of male dignity.

In my experience, most men, when hard, don't act as if their penis is their own, but as if they have suddenly become subject to some kind of erectile radar device that forces them to relinquish all responsibility for its erratic behavior. A-Man, however, presents a complete paradox. Filled with the same juices, the same desires, the same hardness, he never loses his head. He uses his desire to create an event, to push boundaries, to do something not done before. He is the only man I've seen who can walk around a room with a killer erection and still look like a man with a mission—focused, alert, self-contained, and mischievous. He has the most noble erection I've ever met.

Sometimes we discuss just where exactly is his cock going in my body. Somewhere into the center, behind my belly button. We have even measured with the tape measure. Hard to tell the exact angle. What is sure is that he stirs my guts from right to left, forward, upward, sideways, and back. It really gets your attention, having a large cock in your ass, concentrates the mind. Each time, rebirth. Nearly a hundred and fifty so far. That is a lot of starting your whole life over. You might think, after all that ass-fucking, why am I still counting? I'm anal! There you have it. Back to the terrible twos.

The best way to feel, to know, a man's cock is through one's ass, where the walls cling to every inch all the way to the head. A pussy has less feeling, fewer nerves, less strength, less muscular power—and, often, less interest.

A pussy, genetically, wants impregnation, the juice; an asshole wants the ride of its life. Both holes, I would postulate, reconcile the problem of mortality as caverns for creation: vaginas for babies, asses for art.

Speaking of Michelangelo, there is the question of trimming the bush, the male bush. A-Man trims. In the beginning he didn't, and then one day I suggested that a trimmed rim around the base of his cock would look superb, like a samurai warrior. "Depilation is the act of a fastidious lover," states the *Kamasutra.* He thought about it for a minute and then promptly went into the bathroom and sat on the edge of the bathtub. As I held the flashlight, he trimmed. And trimmed, and trimmed. He went far beyond the original idea and just cut down the whole bush—sides, top, balls, underballs, everything. Now there's no going back to the bush. I have much better hand and mouth contact, no little curly hairs in my mouth, and his cock and balls look beautiful. Why doesn't every man trim? Vanity. The hair camouflages their shame. No hair, no shame.

THE LONG AND SHORT OF IT

All this talk about size. From where to where do you measure? From the front side? Belly side? Belly-button side to tip? Or from the base in front of the balls? Or, for that matter, from the more neutral two sides? And then do you measure the penis in a freestanding erection, or can you grasp the base and press down and in toward the body and use that extra inch or so in the measurement? And what are you measuring with? A ruler that doesn't bend? A tape measure that slips? The palm of a hand? A "good eye" combined with a good guess?

And who is doing the measuring? A doctor? A lover? The man on himself? (Can't trust that data.) What with all the possible—and probable—discrepancies, I would say that the calculation of penis size is a most inexact science, a study subject to such extreme variations that when men go on and on and on about size, I don't think they are even comparing penis to penis. In her book *Woman: An Intimate Geography*, Natalie Angier says the average erect human phallus is 5.7 inches (I wonder if she acquired this very precise number from first—or second—hand research? The term *hand job* suddenly takes on new meaning.) Less than half a foot. Yards shorter than a whale's dick, but almost twice the size of a four-hundred-pound gorilla's. God's humor.

Size matters. The perception of size, that is. By the man. In the end, size is more about attitude than inches—but attitude can come with inches. The size of a man's attitude about his penis is more important, and effective, than an extra inch on a small-minded man. On the other hand—or in the same hand, or even both hands—a bigger dick can take a woman farther, farther into herself, deeper into herself. But some women may not wish to go there, be taken there.

How a guy thrusts with his hips is a huge, often overlooked, fucking factor. A small dick with a strong thrust can achieve greater dominance than a big dick that hardly moves, that cannot do the dance. Personally, I cannot love a cock that cannot dominate me. Otherwise I retain too much power. And become totally tyrannical.

And then there's width to consider, something far less frequently referred to by men, which serves to prove yet again that men care more about other men than about their women. A thicker dick can generate an even deeper feeling of domination than a long one—in a pussy, where the most feeling is at the threshold. In an ass, length counts more. Harder to get a long one in, but more profound once there; it feels like it's knocking on your brain as it invades your soul. In short, when it comes to dick size, width for the pussy, length for the ass is the ideal formula . . . which of course underscores the importance of variety. While, obviously, a big cock is not the whole answer—it could of course be attached to an asshole—it can be your hole's answer, which is one place to start.

Women are taught that size doesn't matter, that it's the motion in the ocean. But this is a theory propagated by those bright guys with insecurities who need big theories. The guys who love their dicks are too busy fucking to care. They put their dicks where the others put their theories. Like a good girl, I believed the theory—until I found out I'd been had, not so much by little dicks but by men who thought they had little dicks.

I have learned to be careful with a man who doesn't love his penis. Suspicious of the myriad ways, physical and psychological, that he will compensate. Money, literature, flowers, poetry, promises, proposals, and proficient pussy diving are a few of the camouflages I've been subjected to. But it is always, in the end, a case of the emperor's new clothes, and the insecurity leaks out.

Now, there will always be plenty of women who are happy, happier, with the camouflages. So those men needn't worry—just make sure you get a chick who prefers a real pearl necklace to the washable kind, and a house with a mortgage to your dick in her ass.

I'll admit to penis envy, but only for a big one—if I had one of those, I'd fuck every pretty pussy I could find, nailing each to the cross of her servitude with my big cock. I'd consider it my job, my duty, my destiny. But in the end—in my end, anyway—it is not inches that matter. I have no sense of actual length in my ass, no ruler on my anal walls. I sense size by presence, by pressure, by depth. A-Man is a depth junkie. Of his emotional and spiritual depths I cannot speak with any authority, but I do know that he searches out the depths of my bowels like a demonic Victorian explorer, a gentleman possessed. Like Sir Richard Burton entering Mecca, he is the first Westerner to have infiltrated the tangled jungle of my bowels, my uncharted territory, the heart of my darkness. And he does so with a weapon of singular penetration.

#156

He hangs a large gilt mirror in my bedroom and then I suck his cock in front of it, profile, testing the reflection—it proves worthy. He then sits on the bed and says, "Now just slide back up onto my cock . . ." We're facing the same way. Obedient, I move too fast, too eager, and my ass is pierced with that anal virgin pain. "Okay, okay," he soothes, "I'll do everything . . ."

He turns me over, places me on Pink Square, and rests his cock at the entrance to my ass. Not moving, he reaches around, finds my clit, and pulses her until my ass releases. He then pumps my ass to kingdom come.

THE LESSON

One day we had a conversation. Having discovered how to surrender, I was committed to continue doing so. This entailed remaining
passive, ready to submit, willing to let him manhandle me, to let
him enter my ass. On this particular afternoon, he said that he loved
fucking me—and my ass—that everything was terrific, and if it
stayed as it was, he would still love it. But, he continued, if I learned
how to suck his cock really well, that would be a real bonus. After
swallowing my pride, I said, "Okay, teach me." And he did. So well.
And then I started adding things of my own.

   Sucking a dick is an art form. He gave me some basics. Wet, wet,
wet, the wetter the better. Circling the base above the balls with a
strong grip is good. So is circling the cock and balls with a one-
handed grip. Mouth: no teeth, ever. Smooth, wet, tongue in, or better, tongue long and licking. Then we got to variations of
movement, speed, tension, and rhythm. Change course, he suggested—surprise is good. Don't just do one movement over and
over. Do one movement over and over and then switch. For example: base circled by the thumb-middle-finger cock ring, soft lips

around his cock, down his cock, build up a consistent rhythm, watch his face, see him get closer, then pull out and lick down the back side of his cock, over the balls, and then suction them into your mouth one ball at a time, wet, wet, and with a mouthful of balls roll them around on your tongue like almonds, then lick back up the spine and deep-throat the whole throbbing thing. And variations on this.

Deep is good. Gagging is good. If you won't gag for your man, how can you really love him? Juices more slippery than saliva come up through the throat and coat his cock. It is the throat orgasm.

My blow jobs also made yet another marked improvement in the visual arena, after I sucked his cock in front of several different mirrors. Experimenting with various angles, I learned showmanship, delineation of movement, clarity of intent.

Learning to suck his cock was about concentration. This is the act now, and the only one; it is not a warm-up, it is the main event in that moment. I took these few pointers and practiced, and practiced, and practiced. It's all practice, like ballet, nothing but practice. The more I practiced, the more I discovered, the more I adored his cock, the more I adored myself, the more I adored him, the more I loved sucking his cock, the happier he got. Now he gets so happy that his eyes travel from mine and roll up into his head and his breathing changes and his cheeks flush and I fill with joy like an empty tank at a gas station.

It was while preparing to suck his cock one sunny afternoon that another pillow besides Pink Square found its place. I had been given a tiny, decorative heart-shaped pillow one year for Valentine's Day. It measured only nine inches across, was firmly stuffed, and boasted pink, black, and gold satin stripes on its cover with pink tassels around the circumference. The first time A-Man saw this rather silly little example of female frivolity, he grabbed it in his palm like a football, asked with amused bewilderment, "What's this?," and promptly tossed it off the bed.

He had never seen anything so completely useless being called a pillow; a pillow was for support and comfort, and this particular item promised neither. Until that inspired afternoon when the ostracized little pillow suddenly came into its own. As A-Man sat up at the end of the bed, I grabbed the heart pillow out of his way and, angling the pointed tip toward his ass, placed his balls on it. And there they sat, supported, cock on top, like a royal offering surrounded by shimmering gold threads and dangling pink tassels. We both looked down at the scene in silence. After a brief pause, he announced triumphantly, "It's the Ball Pillow!" We both laughed so hard that his imminent cocksucking was delayed for quite some time. And after that day, he always asked, along with Pink Square, for the Ball Pillow.

He never, ever comes in my mouth. I can suck his cock for forty minutes and he'll hold his power throughout, allowing me to give more, allowing me to love him. Receiving as he does really is a gift to me. I didn't know what a great art cocksucking could be, or what a practitioner I could be, until I found a man who could withstand so much pleasure for such extended lengths of time. So difficult with those guys who come at the mere sight of your mouth on the tip of their cock. It leaves me disabled, impotent.

After I suck his cock more fabulously than ever before, that much deeper, that much slower, that much faster, with a bunch of ball sucking, then, after his eyes roll up into his head several times over and he looks seriously disoriented, he takes my head firmly in his hands, refocuses, looks me straight in the eye and says, "Good girl."

To think I've been through all this, come this far, just to find out that all I ever really wanted was to be a good girl, Daddy's good girl. Finally.

THE UNFORTUNATE
AND BORING PLIGHT OF
SO MANY WOMEN

I am the victim of the unfortunate and boring plight of so many women—Daddy didn't love me enough way back when. And my life with men has become the long trail of my mostly subconscious and sometimes desperate attempts to fill that gap, to feel that love, to heal that hurt, to address that loss. Daddy loves me now, accepts me now, respects me now—and I love him. But this is irrelevant. That hole was dug early and is now part of me. My father can no longer fill it.

Besides, who would I be if he were not my father? Not me. Not me writing this. No, sir. So, in the end, I'm grateful. After all, I wouldn't want to be my unwounded self; she might not like ass-fucking and then where would she be? Certainly not in my privileged position, propped on Pink Square, ass in the air several afternoons a week. She'd probably be doing four loads of laundry for her husband and three children at about that same time and wondering about how to fill that emptiness she feels.

I've only ever met one woman who said that she not only had always adored her father, but that he adored her, always had, and she proudly stated that he was the most beloved man in her life. All the men wanted this woman. She had no hurt, no anger, and no edge. Eventually she married an insanely wealthy entrepreneur. But the rest of us are hurt, angry, and very edgy. Time bombs. Defusing the bomb is a challenge to the feminist man, and arrogance makes him think he can succeed. He can't. It's my hurt, my pain, and who are you to take it from me? I don't need rescuing, I don't need pity, I don't need opinions, I need fucking—and maybe a nice little spanking for indulging my anger.

I have always embraced David Copperfield's challenge to be the heroine of my own life. I just always thought it would involve great public deeds or heart-wrenching sacrifices, but no, it's not like that at all. When I suck his cock and he fucks me in the ass, I am that heroine. It is the deep and sure knowledge that finally, finally, I have really loved a man with no agenda except to love. After my daddy, that is miracle indeed.

He has unwound my wound.

My ass began life as the tiny pale recipient of Daddy's angry hand. It was the place of shame, the site of humiliation, the area to hide from The Hand. It received the proof of my shameful badness, my seemingly unavoidable wrongness. I was Bad and I was Punished. And now that same ass—older but wiser—is the coveted arena of a lover's pleasure where I am naughty and rewarded. And so my ass remains the strongest point of contact with the most important men in my life. It holds my deepest and oldest emotional nerve endings.

Is there a direct connection between getting spanked on the bottom, as I was as a child, and my inclination to being anally penetrated? Possibly. If every father who spanked his little girl thought he might be creating a hungry little sodomite, well, that might be a deterrent.

Being sodomized now, by choice, reconciles this injury with a scenario of the dominant male and the obedient little girl. Instead of rejection and criticism, I am told, "Good girl, good girl." The nastier I am and the better I suck his cock, the better I am, until I'm the goodest little girl in the world. I am finally loved. The relief it brings me is profound.

I, with my total submission, in fact wield a great healing power: the more I submit the more excited he gets, until I enter the deepest phase of surrender and he comes. He only comes when I've given it up. It takes a lot of surrender, discipline, and love to let a man fuck your ass hard enough, long enough, deep enough, and fast enough to shoot. His orgasm is my victory over my lesser self, over the pain of my anger. It fills the hole; I'm finally whole.

#162

Owwww! My dad just left after a lovely friendly visit of a week, and three hours later I was doubled over in literal gut-wrenching pain lasting a solid twenty-four hours. Like I'd been punched in the stomach, like I'd rewound in one hour 161 unwinding ass fucks. So the only logical thing to do was go for #162. Jesus, that hurt. New levels of tolerance, new levels of release, new levels of discipline. As he entered I thought, not so painful, I'm already healed by being naked with my ass on display. I was wrong. By the time he got in five inches and then some, he was pushing into the fist in my gut and rolfing me from the inside. It hurt like hell but I didn't say a word. I just maintained the pain level just past bearable and adored the challenge all the while thinking, Girl, you really are Daddy's little masochist.

DEVOTION

A-Man does not require my devotion, he says, but he has it anyway. Sometimes I give up so much power to him, give up even more than I have, and this leaves me vulnerable just beyond my own capacity to endure. The best antidote for this is not biting the bullet and suffering like some deeply ethical woman—I have, at least, matured beyond that. No, the antidote is another guy. It's called "The Two-Guy Solution." Every woman should subscribe when necessary. Many already do without admitting to it. As one friend put it, "If you're having trouble with one man, just call another man." For me, A-Man with the occasional Hound form the ideal combination. Someone needs to give to me as I give to him—power, that is.

While it is my greatest desire to surrender to him, with anyone else I am dominant. I never fuck anyone else, and no one else goes in my ass with their cock.

On one occasion, shortly after #169, I felt the need and called an old Hound friend. He announced, to my surprise, that he really wanted to fuck me—which was out of the question. But he let it be known that for a price he would eat my pussy: amazing how demanding Hounds can get when left alone too long. The money would give him detachment—he would be a tongue for hire. I loved the idea of turning a man into a whore—though it did feel a little too politically correct. But before even negotiating a price, he proposed that he would give me a freebie under the condition that I be entirely dominant, dictating every turn, every move, fulfilling my every desire. Okay, okay, I said—but just this once. I can, on occasion, be compliant with a Hound; I could be a dominatrix for a night. It would, however, have been easier to pay him. We were now both "topping from the bottom"—and I wasn't sure who was actually in charge anymore.

He came over and I was ready for him, reclining on my bed in my boudoir in black lingerie. First I asked for admiration while he sat in a chair. Why was I the hottest chick at the party? He explained. In his life? He explained further. I found this game to be quite fun. In the whole world? He explained still further, but this time I was not convinced. Next game. We examined my ass in the mirror from all angles, and he pointed out every curve and line to explain why it was the best ass—best in the boudoir, anyway. Then we looked at how my shaved pussy lips peeked through my thighs below my ass when I bent over. This was really fun—right out there with it all, shamelessly.

So far he hadn't been allowed to touch me. Lying on my bed, I then asked for a back massage, then a breast and stomach massage, then a butt massage, then a hip and thigh massage. Then I told him to go back to the chair, sit down, take out his cock, and stroke himself while I displayed my pussy to him like a stripper girl on the runway, spread lips, swollen red clit, long lean legs, killer shoes. He got pretty fucking hard.

Then I asked that he lick my pussy for a while, taking long strokes from my ass to my pussy to my clit and back again, the whole wet package. That was great. Really just great. Next I asked him to concentrate on rimming my asshole with slowly increasing pressure until his tongue started forcing its way inside: "Like you want it." "Like?" He did want it. Then he served me four or five inches of a red chili pepper vibrator up my ass. I hadn't asked for that part, so to speak, but it was hot so I didn't object.

Then followed some straight-on clit licking, for as long as it took while I tried to hold out. During this time I indulged all my fantasies, flipping randomly through my Rolodex. Of A-Man watching this other guy lick me and being amused at my outrageous indulgence, approving, and saying to him: "You keep doing that till she's had enough, then I'll fuck her ass." Then I fantasized that A-Man was licking my clit relentlessly—but that was way too exciting, so I had to stop. Then I imagined all the men I've been with, and dumped, in a lineup, outside my bedroom window, watching. I displayed my pleasure and my juice like a whore. On and on with the fantasies until the final one, the finishing one: Reality.

This man, for reasons I don't really understand—could it be love?—is willing to be slave to my orgasm, licking until I have had enough (and enough for me, of course, is a lot). This overwhelming experience of abundance pushed me, unexpectedly, into a state of gratitude that manifested in a full body, curved, deep, silent orgasm that took twenty minutes to return from. The Hound, dear, darling Hound, left me quietly, so I could bask in the enormity of the blessedness of my life and the peace of power returned: his submission to me balancing mine to A-Man. Now I'm ready to be fucked in the ass again. I'll do whatever it takes to be ready for A-Man. This is a measure of my devotion — and, I suppose, of the Hound's, too.

RAZING THE BAR

Training as a classical ballet dancer, as I did, is surely the most intense physical training possible for a young body—day in, day out, hour after hour of meticulous sculpting, shaping, and coercing the body, the belly, and the limbs into shapes, angles, and lines that reach far, far beyond one's natural physical state. Always going for more of everything, more length, more turns, more turnout, more strength, more-more-more. It takes both body and mind into a place of existence that is beyond normal experience. I learned from the age of four to experience my life through my body, inside my body, always on the brink of perpetual endurance.

All this, I believe, prepared me for getting fucked in the ass. It answers the call of my physical masochism. It re-creates the physical extremism of dancing, the discipline, the striving for perfection. It is my being in extremis. Now that I am retired from dancing all of life has a dull edge—except this. A-Man calls it "the Hard Edge of Truth."

Dancing is about being in service to the choreographer, to the steps, to the music. Allowing this man into my ass reproduces this dynamic of service, of yielding to something greater than myself. Learning to go past—way past—one's physical comfort level, and to love that moment of going past, is intrinsic to a dancer's training. It is only in passing this place that one finds that Edge where Risk is real and Rapture resides.

If you have a ballerina's tight ass like mine, the pain and pleasure of the internal pressure of sodomy are inseparable. Ballet school perfects the desire to be perfect, and you can end up a delightful and disciplined little slave. I understand that receiving a cock in your ass goes right in tandem with the psychology of perfectionism that afflicts high achievers like myself. To begin with, we need it: being perfect results in a very tight ass. Secondly, the challenge to remain perfect while being anally penetrated is one of the greatest challenges one could entertain. To succeed surely proves one's inner and outer perfection of being, shape, health, and resilient attitude. Recipient sodomy is a perfectionist's dream, a masochist's nirvana.

But—as with most things anal—the opposite is also true. Getting ass-fucked while wearing one's metaphorical tutu is perhaps the ballerina's most propitious—and scandalous—debut. But it is also her crucifixion, her ultimate sacrifice to transcend the human to find the divine. Never on the stage, however, did I feel as safe as I do when I obey A-Man completely and he covers my face with his big, strong hand and rocks my ass onto his cock. An incredible sense of relief—I have completely let go not only of all control but all responsibility and have given it to him. The sense of safety is so high with him because any time spent with him is the only waking time when my anxiety is gone, when I am not afraid.

#175

Well, I did just give him a truly insane blow job—cock, balls, ass-hole—the full run over and over, ending every now and then with full cock-throat immersion. Every blow job for me is an act of insanity because I feel every one could be the last, and so every one contains all I have. Fuck on the edge. Suck on the edge. All ways.

OLD ORGASMS

Is anal sex sex? I keep on wondering about this. My connection to him is primarily penetrative and, specifically, anal. Is this sex? Or merely an act of spiritual submission, divine submission?

My orgasm arc with him is an act of giving, opening, giving. With others it is withholding, a battleground of control. In the past, I have achieved orgasm through the paradoxical experience of maintaining control of my pleasure all the while that my orgasm, with a life force of its own, desires its own fruition. The battle—and it is a battle—always ends with an orgasm more potent for its release than for any emotional pleasure. There are quite a few men out there who want nothing more than to please. For them I come in angry triumph: the greater my contempt for their wishing-to-please, the greater my resistance; the greater my resistance, the greater my orgasm. This is the pleasure, literally—and clitorally—of the war between the sexes. Afterwards, so sensitized, I shun all touch and, like Garbo, want to be alone. To take notes, eat dinner, and read *The New Yorker*. Is this any way to come? Well, it is one way.

With him I have learned another. The way of no resistance. Of infinite contractions and many arrivals. And it was not a struggle to give up the struggle. It just happened with him, as if my body knew—I sure didn't—that he was the one, the one man I could trust, the one man I could give to without his misinterpreting the gift, taking advantage of it, making it mean what it didn't mean. Perhaps it was his beauty. DNA to DNA. He does have, objectively speaking, the most beautiful physique of them all. Maybe my clit knew he was my sexual mate long before I did. Just as it knew that resistance was necessary to all those men whose DNA was not a match for mine. With them I come from hostility, with him from love.

#181

Last night—181.

I tell him, after, "A hundred and eighty-one." And I point out that that is just ass-fucks, that does not count pussy warm-ups.

"What does that tell you?" I say.

"That tells me three-hundred and sixty-two," he said, "that's what that tells me. Three sixty-two tells me it's a good year."

SOUVENIRS

As we approached two hundred, I found that my desire for continual repetition, for impossible guarantees, was intensifying. Managing my relentless need to be in that place with him became a full-time job. There was the disastrous day when the cleaning lady grabbed his well-worn shirt off my bed with the sheets and I came home and saw, to my horror, that she had washed, dried, and neatly folded my aromatic lifeline. I had slept every night with the shirt that smelled like him. Now it smelled like Bounce.

All these endless words thrown toward this act, this Holy Fuck, all in the attempt to believe it, believe in something so deep and powerful, to hold on to it, to not let it expire into the black hole of my private terror. My demons are like an infection in the soul and they desire to devour and destroy the truth—and even the beauty—of my very own experience. They are the Devils. My Devils. Damn the Devils.

It's all about evidence. My quest for evidence. Evidence of attachment because attachment predicts repetition. Once one has been taken to the land of primal joy, revisiting that land becomes one's sole desire. Words, a call, a look, a sigh, the third erection of the afternoon, all are evidence. A condom shot through with cum; two condoms, one shot through with cum, the other empty because he pulled out and shot up my back and into the soft hair at the nape of my neck. His worn shirt, his scent—my madeleine. Or it can be a fuck count. That is why I count, to know it really happened, to know it might happen again. Like a detective, I amass the evidence of love, love that was, love that is, and therefore try to convince my internal jury that love will be. All too often, however, I don't believe the evidence. Until the next time. Another number, another reprieve. Another shot, another high.

I am an anal addict, but only with him. I want it consistently, frequently, repetitively, ritually, and if I don't get it I become sad, tearful, lonely, beleaguered, unhappy, grouchy, faithless, and miserable. I want to mainline him. Only his penetration of my ass excavates my fear and restores my faith, the faith he created.

When an experience of love arrives that demotes all others to impostors, it brings, inside the joy, a haunting fear. How could this delight have been showered upon me, a mortal woman with the usual sins, unhealed wounds, desperate anger, and fierce desire?

"Why me?" says my voice of disbelief.

"Why not me?" says a small, faint voice not my own, echoing up from my gut.

Then I found the best evidence of all—the one that actually worked, that relieved the withdrawal symptoms and gave me solace. He had a game, the postcoital fling-the-condom-into-the-wastebasket-by-the-bed game. Not surprisingly, his aim was amazingly accurate. After he left, I would resituate the condom so that it dangled over the top edge of the basket, the pocket of cum weighing it down, the rim secured by the still sticky K-Y. And I would leave this trophy there where I could easily see it, until the next time he called and said, "It's Time." Time to shave my pussy, time to turn off the phone, time to make way for new DNA, time for time to end. With this ritual I contrived to never be without his molecular makeup near me at all times.

Whenever I looked at that condom, and I looked a lot, I felt the rush of his beauty. I've always been a sucker for symbolism; this dangling rubber provided me with the opaque evidence of what was, and will be again. I clung to his DNA until given the next deposit— as if my subconscious took refuge in the theoretical knowledge that there was a possibility at all times of re-creating his essence. Those condoms comforted me, reminding me of the fourth dimension, the dimension beyond bills, anxiety, self-loathing, and desire, the dimension where bliss reigns, and I am its babbling slave.

#200

Always before, I doubt.

   Always after, I don't.

   Two hundred entries into my bowels, two hundred times I doubt and then believe.

   What's it going to take? Two hundred and one.

FOREPLAY

Knock . . . knock . . . knock. When I open the front door, he is always slow to enter. He is in no rush; A-Man knows where he's going. And where he's coming, too. He steps inside, I lock the door, and we are sealed inside together. I feel the warmth rising already. Then the hug, the holding. The full-body holding that starts the coming, his and mine. Strong, enveloping, possessive. I start moaning and I feel his cock pushing at me. He grabs my hips and presses them into, onto, his cock. It's hard to break the hug, but we must get to the bedroom; it's imperative. If we don't make it there, tchotchkes always get smashed. The bedroom is our padded cell, where insanity can be unleashed without excessive material damage.

Sometimes he just turns me around, facing forward, his cock pressed up against my ass, and keeping the contact, leads me to the bedroom as we synchronize our walk so as not to break position. But before the first step, I find my speaking voice, and ask if he wants any food, if he's hungry. He always declines, but I always ask. We are very polite with each other.

Once we're in the bedroom, the hug is often revisited. Those first hugs establish Loveland, but now it's time to leave that invisible place and travel to Lustland, where things are visible and tangible and so unreal. Now he's totally hard, his pants aren't fitting right at all. He backs away from me and slowly, carefully, deliberately takes off all his clothes, keeping his eyes on me the whole time. I just watch and wait. He'll let me know what he wants. He always does.

Sometimes he'll speak softly and say, "Get on the bed — on your knees — now pull up your dress." Then he eats me out, from behind. Other times, he will just take my body and position me where he wants me — crouching on a pillow before him as he feeds me his cock, or flat on my back on the bed while he pinches my nipples through my dress or . . . But whatever happens now, it's all in slow motion. After a lot of cocksucking, and I mean a lot, he moves me around and grabs a condom and then I know we are about to enter the next stage.

Pussy sex is foreplay. Sometimes he skips my pussy altogether and goes straight to my ass, really nasty, only ass — the exit stage. But usually he does pussy first. As he enters me I feel him push up against my cervix, push into my cervix, and it always startles me. I enter the Zone of Release. Sometimes he'll get so far up there and then start pulsing, with expert little thrusts, pushing my walls outward, upward, further into my being. Every pulse wants more and gets more. This is the beginning of moreness, a state of body longing that craves without cease. The waves of pleasure roll in slowly, then more quickly, but they never stop. Pinnacle after pinnacle, most might deem it the best ever, even transcendent. But he and I are greedy and know where to go for more. There is this amazing moment where love is saturating the room and yet loss is not present. We're just beginning. Just warming up.

After he has had enough pussy (always his choice), he pulls out and situates me—sometimes on Pink Square, sometimes on all fours, sometimes sideways, hip curved upward like a Henry Moore. However he sees it, he gets it. Already well fucked, I am now at my most obedient. My will is now about 40 percent depleted, but I am still holding on to my consciousness, to my awareness, and to my high heels. I have much more to give. Much more. I have the power to give, give power. Other lovers never even got 10 percent of what I have to give. They didn't have the power to ask for it. He does . . . and then he asks for more than that.

REAR ENTRY

He places me on my left side, two pillows snug under my hip, raising my ass in a fetching little upward sideways arch. I rest my left cheek on the bed, turn my head, and look up to him — it's always up with him, never down. He grabs one of the tubes of K-Y scattered about the bed. I adore the sound as the top clicks open. Looking at me, he squeezes a gob onto two of his fingers. Looking to my ass, he spreads my cheeks so deliberately I cannot believe my luck. He rubs the gel gently, firmly onto my asshole, into my asshole, rimming the entryway, smoothing the passage. There is the most wondrous look on his face as he does this, alternately gazing in my eyes and gazing to my ass. He slips a finger inside, then two, watching my face, keeping the gaze as I feel his fingers turning inside me, connecting us internally and externally, full circle. Sliding his fingers out, he squeezes more K-Y onto his fingers and rubs it smoothly along the length of his cock, hard as a rock.

It's Time.

Holding his cock, he guides it toward the crack in my ass, like a canoe aiming down a narrow ravine. I feel the smooth tip, both hard and velvety on my skin. The center of my asshole, like a magnet, gravitates toward the pressure. We meet. His key to my door, his positive to my negative, his plug to my socket.

And the light goes on.

Center to center, he nudges, I breathe, he pushes, I release, he pulses, I open, he pushes, he pushes, I open, he plunges in, our eyes lock, and he sends me home.

Sometimes he'll then pull back, and thrust short at the entry for a while, other times he'll slide inward, downward, slowly, slowly until he is buried in my ass with no cock to spare, only balls outside. He'll stay there for a moment, not moving. Then he'll pulse farther. Sometimes he will move me into a different position—on my hands and knees; or standing up while bending over, hands plastered to the wall; or on my back, feet to the ceiling; or, a favorite, legs over my head and ass to the ceiling. Whichever position I'm in, he remains above me, always looking down upon me, watching me, loving me. And he'll usually make these shifts without pulling his dick from my ass. Totally fantastic. But whatever the angle I can feel his cock growing inside me, stronger, harder, deeper, pressing into my anxieties, my pettiness, my pride, my vanity. Like a vacuum to dust, he sucks out my lesser selves, removes my sins. One by one they are suctioned away and underneath he finds my goodness, my innocence, my four-year-old before she was hit by The Hand and got mad. This is what he was looking for. This is what he finds. This is what he gives me.

Fucked off my feet, my shoes fall to the floor with a thud, one by one. He smiles and says affectionately, "Now we're having fun." Now I'm traveling on the fast train to paradise. Unschooled as I am in the process, tears often fall out of my eyes. Like a true gentleman, he will shield my eyes with his broad hand, giving me privacy, while he fucks me harder and harder, faster and faster, squeezing out the tears.

When I finally release everything, not one centimeter of my being holding on to anything at all, when my ego is annihilated, then the laughing begins. It can begin while I'm still crying, the energies are the same, though the tears are more familiar. But somewhere, somehow, along the way, my unconscious bursts open and I laugh and laugh and laugh. The harder I laugh the harder he fucks my ass until the whole thing makes no sense at all. Now we are really having fun. He looks at me laughing, and then, content that I'm on the road with him, he fucks me some more, ever vigilant, ever present. My laugh sometimes deepens and I laugh like I never laughed before. I recognized it immediately the first time it happened—the cackle of the crone. It is the sound of a woman who is caught inside the mystery of the universe, in the irony of the angst, in the place that ego abhors. Bliss.

At first the pleasure was unbearable and I'd try to pull away, try to know what was happening. But he doesn't let me, fucking me so relentlessly that any attempt to backtrack to control is useless. It is here that his domination is complete. I am his slave and he forces harmony upon me, against my ferocious fear. With repetition I have come to accept it, and now I don't only visit but have learned how to stay there. Meanwhile he is looking at me, all tears, giggles, and gut-laughs, and says, "You are CRAZY, girl." He looks a little dazed himself, but unlike me, he maintains total control, total awareness.

I look up as he kneels above me, deep inside me, and I see the most beautiful thing I ever saw. Like Michelangelo's *David*, his chest is broad, his skin is smooth, his hands are huge, his face beatific. I see the beauty of this man, the beauty of man.

I never saw this before.

#220

I fell madly, quickly, and completely, forever, the first time he fucked my ass. Now it's #220 and my love has only deepened—220 times deeper. I adore him, for good and better (it's never worse), and it is a kind of rapturous indulgence to so unconditionally adore the entire skin surface of another human being's body. Before I liked men in parts—their lips or eyes, their hands or chest, only occasionally the cock itself. With him I love all those and every nook, cranny, and space in between—and his cock, balls, and asshole most of all.

In worship lies freedom. The freedom of withholding nothing, which propels one into the elliptical realm of love.

ANAL ORGASM

As I learned how to stay in the bliss, I found something else. I have become pure vehicle for his cock, no resistance. I can relinquish all power. I feel such a gravitational pull to this man, who can, and will, disempower me, so willing to give everything away, to bestow it upon him. I never knew how much power I had until I gave it all to him through my ass. My ass is a pipeline for power.

I am, I have come to realize, his runway, his launchpad. And after numerous runs to the edge of inevitability, the final one begins. I can tell it's the one because it coincides, always, with my ability to commit to complete submission, to remain completely open without reserve, without limit. Once he feels this, he aims for the gold. If I show any sign on my face, or inside my ass, of reneging on my submission, he slows down and works me until my ass believes that there is only one choice, only one way. No choice but surrender is surrender. I am his entirely, body, soul, and asshole. I relish my freedom.

Molded onto his cock, I feel its urgency. The road to orgasm is a straight line into my ass, into the center of my being, into the center of the world. I don't know who starts the coming. I do, however, know that he is the only man whose orgasm interests me more than my own—no small feat. On one level, I feel like his cock sets off my contractions and my contractions then set off his . . . but then his set off mine . . . Contractions in my ass, involuntary contractions: anal orgasm.

I ride his orgasm like a jockey on a wild stallion, never losing contact but never in control. He explodes. My ass has sucked us together into an airless vacuum and we are one thing. Fused in a timeless space, I experience my destiny directly as being that moment and no other.

We are very happy after. We usually don't speak, just eyes in eyes. I used to like discussing the event once I regained my voice. What is it? What is it really about? Why does it happen? What, in fact, is happening? On and on. We don't discuss it now, because I know I shall never really understand. Now I am just grateful. Now I just want a three-hour ass-fuck where I give him all my power, he takes it, and takes me to visit God. That's all I need. Over and over and over. I want to die with him in my ass.

#246

Last night I am home from a three-week trip. He is over, and we are silent. He fucks my mouth and my pussy both, long and hard. Then, in my newly virgin ass, slow, deep, one plunge to the hilt. When all in, with my ass suctioning about his cylinder, he finally speaks. "Welcome home."

"Welcome home," I echo, sucking him in.

Later, tired, jet-lagged, overwhelmed, I start to cry—though nothing is particularly wrong. He looks at me weeping and tells me how wonderful my life is and then places my clenched little hand over his crotch, saying, "And I've got this big cock here for you— you can hold it if you like." I break from my self-pity and grab in his shorts, finding his cock in the folds, the gearshift that drives my life. I look up to his face in the shadows and see his eyes are glistening. Then a drop runs slowly down his cheek . . . and another. Astonished, I ask why he is crying. "I don't know," he murmurs. Almost 250 ass-fucks got us here, into the essence of unspoken sweetness.

THE BOX

A beautiful, tall, round, hand-painted Chinese lacquered box. Black and gold. Shiny. A pussycat with long white whiskers on the lid.

The collection.

The collection of the collection.

The condoms. Used. Filled. Hundreds.

Latex, sealed with K-Y.

Evidence. My mortality. His immortality.

DNA. The X and the Y. The Code. Forever.

My homage.

My altar.

My treasure.

His life.

PARADISE

I have learned a few things, by now, about Paradise.

Paradise is not that thing in the nebulous, far-off future, in another place, or another world, or another galaxy. It is not a state of mind, or a place in the mind. Nor is it the exquisite sexual pleasure of pulsing blood and moaning desire. Paradise is not achieved only after great suffering. There may well be great suffering before or after Paradise, but it is not the requirement for entry. Wounded ego and rampant narcissism demand suffering. Paradise is just there, here, if you really want it.

I am sitting on the threshold. Perhaps this is the final paradox of God's paradoxical machinations: my ass is my very own back door to heaven. The Pearly Gates are closer than you think. Sacred and profane united in one hole.

Paradise is free. A gift. A state of grace. A dance of time and space. It resides inside the ego and outside the ego, a place of pure harmony, another body riding your ass like it was the last fuck on earth.

Paradise is an experience that in real time may last only seconds.

But in those immeasurable fragments, time stops, and only when time stops does death die and Paradise is entered. It is revealed in the spaces of time when the self is penetrated so deeply that it is pried wide open and love rushes in like an ocean through a porthole.

And Paradise, once known, becomes the goal of every waking moment, its loss inherent in every waking moment. This is the burden of Paradise found.

#262

He's back! He was gone but now he's back. A phone call and he's over. Declarations. Tears. Hilarity. Clarity. In front of the blazing fire, insane kissing, sucking, and fucking. Insane. Completely insane.

I am clear. Clearly blinded. I am his mother, sister, daughter, and friend. He is my father, brother, son, and friend.

After, we watch the flames and he says, "See what we've done?"

"What?"

"We've created love out of sex . . . And we've only just begun."

"Yeah," I say, "Maybe I'll fuck you in the ass next."

He grins, pauses, and tells me to stand in front of him, turn around . . . and he bends me over . . .

No dice with A-Man.

REAR-ENDED

Where do you go once in Paradise? What happens when Adam and Eve enter Eden? And eat the apple? I will tell you. Perfection cannot be maintained. With time, cracks appear in the walls of the Garden—and reality, insipid reality, slithers in with its insidious poison. The snake of knowledge.

At some point well past the two-year mark, my relentless attempts to trust that A-Man was real and really in my life paid off. I had finally convinced myself that there was some form of unpredictable continuity to our connection. Before, I had only one focus: the need to believe in our existence. But once I finally accepted "reality," the rest of the world soon followed. I tried to plug the leaks, ignore the signs, deny the chaos—but the world proved to be even stronger than my passion for A-Man.

He was constantly leaving town for work; sometimes for weeks, sometimes for months. I found his absences increasingly difficult to manage. One time, I hired a pretty woman in a pink-sequined minidress to come to my house and pray for me, while I cried, for a hundred and fifty dollars. That's how bad it was.

Then he called. Prayer answered. All's well, he says, except one thing. His cock won't reach across four states into my ass. Things are funny and good again, for a few hours. And I don't tell him just how difficult things are for me. Never told him. Ever. Why would I? Reality was oozing in anyway, but why open the door wide?

Another time I consulted with a friend, afraid that after his three-month absence he wouldn't return to me as before. My friend laughed: "Two-hundred and sixty-something ass-fucks and you need more evidence?" The only one that counts, I explain, is the next one. And I am dead serious. I then explored a sex and love addiction twelve-step program, went to a few meetings, and read the textbook. From its point of view—which I tried adopting for a week or so—he is my drug, I am an addict, and abstinence is the beginning of re-covery. This information was horrifying—my situation was an ill-ness! And comforting—I could follow their plan to heal from this illness, in the company of similarly sick people, and get all the sup-port I wanted.

But I was assailed by doubts. When is it love and when is it ad-diction? Did I, once again, want to pathologize myself, especially af-ter my hard-won sexual liberation? Did I wish to regard the great opening of my heart and ass as a problem to be solved rather than a gift to be honored? Did I wish to view this flawed, flesh-and-blood man as nothing but a projection of my own illusions, obsessions, conflicts, and screaming sexual desires? This felt like a limited per-spective. Besides, the first thing a sex addict must do is to stop hav-ing sex. I'd suffered celibacy in my ten-year marriage; was I now going to choose it voluntarily? The textbook had a whole chapter on just what hell to expect from withdrawal — I found little solace in it. It would be hell indeed to withdraw from loving whom I loved. Perhaps this was not the pain of an addict in the grip of disease but simply the pain of a woman in love confronted with the loss of her beloved. (When I told A-Man, much later, after #270, that I was "addicted" to him, he looked highly amused and responded without missing a beat, "You damn well better be.")

There were other disincentives to "recovery." The meetings were mostly attended by men with a lot of compulsive-masturbation and Internet-porn obsessions. I imagined their computer monitors stained with crusty semen drips and their sexual fantasies running wild as they shared their distraught and ambivalent hopes of abstinence. It felt dangerous to be an attractive woman in their presence. Then, at the end of one meeting, a reforming addict held my hand with just a little too much sympathy and I never went back. My problem was love; his was lechery.

I then turned to Buddhist meditation to deconstruct my suffering — to accept it as a karmic consequence of my past lives and present life, to tolerate it without blaming anyone, even to welcome it as part of life's natural cycle. I tried to look at my own contribution to my unhappiness. I would meditate on the suffering of others, and attempt to lay the groundwork for less suffering of my own the next time he left town. I would try to remember that the pain of my loss and attachment is an illusory phenomenon.

I thought about how simple life might be if one removed sexuality from the equation. Between the search, the conquest, the fucking itself, the residual emotions, and the desire for repetition, my sex life was almost a full-time job: without it, I could save a great deal of time and energy. A very great deal. For what? Compassion for all rather than obsession with one?

But after months and months of all this "spiritual" work, I still wanted A-Man in my ass—as frequently and as predictably as possible. I was, it appeared, incurable.

There I was—searching, searching, searching for the solution to my pain to no avail. Then she found me.

HER

One day, walking into the locker room at the gym, I saw the quiet brunette, the one I assumed A-Man fucked on occasion. I said my usual warm hello, but instead of her usual warm smile back, I was greeted with an icy stare and sulky silence.

The next time I saw A-Man, I recounted the exchange. Did he know why she might have snarled at me? Well, yes, he did know. Apparently she had recently confronted him, demanding to be told if he was fucking anyone besides her. (Surely, I thought smugly to myself, she already knew the answer to that particular question.) He said that he asked her if she was certain she wanted an answer, and she insisted that she did. So he said yes. But she didn't stop there. She wanted to know who. So he told her about me. Apparently this was a total surprise to her. She had known we were friends, but I guess she didn't know the whole of it. Or the half of it. Or the back half of it. Well, he told me, she couldn't stop crying. He clearly didn't feel good about this, but he also knew that he'd only told her what she'd insisted on hearing.

Was she sorry, I wondered, that she'd asked? It seemed like such an obvious error on her part. She was not, apparently, only snarling at me, but very angry at him as well. I was slower to realize that I, too, had asked about something better left alone; if I had never queried him about my encounter with the mousy brunette, A-Man would never have mentioned their blowup. It was us women asking for information that we didn't really want that precipitated the events that followed. On that day, however, I just listened, feeling somewhat aloof. If anything, I enjoyed that slight thrill of drama in our midst as we proceeded into the glory of ass-fuck #272.

But the next day, and the one after that, I realized that I had been given unsolicited confirmation that he *was* fucking her on occasion and I really hadn't wanted to know that. This made her real to me in a way that she never had been before. Were we competing for A-Man? She clearly thought so, and was putting up some sort of fight, or at least a protest. I had always assumed that there was no fight, no competition, because I was simply in the far superior position to her or anyone else that A-Man might have been fucking. It was technically impossible that he could have been having anything greater or even equivalent with anyone else—there simply wasn't time in a day, or cum in his balls . . . Or was there?

And thus my mind started working. What was their connection? How was their sex? Was he with her the way he was with me? Did he mold her onto his cock the way he did me? Did her fuck her ass, too? What had he done to make her so attached? And what about her kept his interest? Was she to him what a Hound was for me—a balancing act? Now that his little harem was in my face, I couldn't pretend it wasn't there. The jealousy began and I couldn't stop it. But I was determined to try.

This, I reminded myself, was the price of not being monogamous. Perhaps it was time to review the price of monogamy.

If I asked A-Man to be monogamous, then I would always know I had taken his freedom, and I loved him basking in his freedom. I did not want to control him. I remembered him saying once, "You go out with a chick, you sleep with her once, and she hands you an armful of 'do nots,' and you're looking at her great tits and her hot pussy and you're looking at the 'do nots' in your arms and you hand them back. 'Hey, I think these are yours.'" I had admired that— that's why he was A-Man and not Any Man. He was not going to compromise himself for pussy, like so many men do. And I didn't want to compromise a man with my pussy, I wanted a man to be true to himself . . . while desperately wanting my pussy.

But this was only idle speculation, for I knew that A-Man would not be monogamous, even if I asked. He had told me long ago that he had tried being a boyfriend several times and always failed miserably. Better not to even try. I agreed. Failure is the great anti-aphrodisiac.

Besides, if I wanted him to be only with me then I would have to return the favor and be only with him. And I knew that I couldn't do that. I loved him too much. I was too vulnerable to give myself entirely to him. Without a commitment that might be broken, at least any pangs I might be feeling about the mousy brunette were not compounded by the self-righteous pain and anger of betrayal.

So, I told myself, Do you know what you have to be if you're not monogamous? Not jealous? No, jealousy is inevitable. Worth it. You've got to be worth it. He's got to be worth it. The fucking has got to be worth it. Worth the occasional, gut-ripping insanity of jealousy.

WAR

As the days passed, however, I started feeling this overwhelming need to assert my authority over the mousy brunette. When I next saw A-Man I slyly suggested that we all get in bed together to assuage everyone's pain with love and sperm. He smiled at me, loving that I was the kind of woman who would solve a problem with an orgy. Well, better than bayonets. He then said that he had actually suggested this to her during that first confrontation but that she had only cried harder in response, confessing that she would be too jealous. Damn. I knew if we could get her in bed, I could win. Suddenly winning became imperative. Winning what, exactly, I wasn't sure, but the stakes seemed very high indeed. It was not about having him exclusively, it never had been; it was about knowing I was the most beloved.

It subsequently became completely imperative for me to distinguish myself from her in my own mind. A-Man had told me that she'd had affairs with married men in the past; I decided that she must have a history of playing second fiddle to other women. Whereas I, on the other hand, am always lead masochist, head girl, first-best, or I don't play. Period. I also became inordinately, insanely fixated on the size of her ass. It was, after all, twice mine, if not more . . . maybe two and half times mine . . . If A-Man so loved my tight ass, how could he love that wide one, too?

Then, a few weeks later, we all had the misfortune to overlap at the gym. Having finished my own exercise routine, I was leaving through the check-in area and there they both were, sitting on the couch: she was scowling, and he looked as if he'd rather be anywhere else. What had happened to the sex god who strode about my bedroom with the killer erection? This man pulled his legs under him on the couch and stared at his knees, barely breathing.

I breezed through on my way out the door, saying a bright hello to both. What else could I do? And while I didn't expect her to respond, I was, I realize, testing him. And he failed me. Silence. No acknowledgment of me in front of her. Outside, devastated, I burst into tears. I needed something from him and I wasn't getting it. And I wasn't going to get it. Assurance. But of course—and this was the catch-22 that lay at the core of our whole affair—had he given me the assurance I so desperately needed, of my place in his hierarchy and his heart, the fire between us would most likely have been extinguished. It was always just the right balance of that element of not being sure that kept me so in love, so full of desire, so very excited about him. He had never bent to my will, and that wasn't going to change now. He had always shown me his love; but he wouldn't confirm it on demand.

∽

It was clear to me that A-Man was going to do nothing to resolve this problem. So I had to do something. I got this idea in my head to discuss with the mousy brunette, in a girlie kind of way, the problem, our problem: him. This woman's agony was now threatening the safety of my world with A-Man, and perhaps if we talked, she and I could work something out. Besides, it wasn't just her pain anymore; it was also mine. The story was becoming about her and me, with A-Man watching from the sidelines. Was this some unresolved Electra thing? Maybe, but I had no time to think about mythology right now. This was war. And, with her, I had no intention of surrendering.

Contriving to run into her at the gym, I approached her boldly in my carefully planned outfit and asked if we had "something to talk about." Although she was not sure that we did, she said she was willing to talk. I asked her what had happened. She said that she had been so unhappy with him, with having so little of him, that she'd asked him about the other women in his life. The Truth Will Set You Free Strategy: she'd suspected that his answer would hurt her, but she'd hoped that it would give her the courage to stop seeing him.

Well, clearly it hadn't, because almost immediately she was trying the same strategy again with me, asking me all these intensely personal questions. How often did he and I fuck? Did he sleep over? Did we eat dinner together? And I found myself doing the most awful thing. I found myself answering her, praying that this time her strategy would succeed, even though I knew it wouldn't.

And so we all limped along: no monogamy, no threesome, more fucking, no resolution.

#276

He directed me onto all fours. He stood behind me and gently but insistently tapped my pubic bone skyward. I raised my ass to meet him. He tapped the insides of both thighs. I separated my legs. I laid my head down on the bed, ass high, back arched. He parted my pussy, found my little clit, and began looking and sucking and flicking. I imagined that other chick, the one with the wide ass, sitting in a chair, naked, legs spread, as he knelt before her pussy. Not an ugly pussy, but a bigger pussy than mine, a different, mousy pussy, and as she sat slumped, spread and slutty, he sucks on her clit, her obvious, swollen, big red clit. She is uninvolved, shameless. I am watching this secretly from behind a door. He knows I'm watching and spreads her pussy more and more so I can see her clit. She doesn't know I'm watching. As her clit stands out, like a small erect cock, proud, flagrant, and hungry, I come. Conquest of the other woman is my orgasm, my pleasure. The other woman is my whore—the whore in me. Then he fucks my pussy and then my ass. My clit runneth over.

THE BANANA

The memory of humiliation is the bleeding scar of reliving it. . . . Humiliation, I believe, is not just another experience in our life, like, say, an embarrassment. It is a formative experience. It forms the way we view ourselves as humiliated persons.

—AVISHAI MARGALIT

Funny—well, not really—how I began to lose the ability to receive pleasure directly from A-Man but had to siphon it through another woman, his other woman. So sexy in bed, so catastrophic out of bed. And thus I erected yet another Freudian triangle as I fantasized pulling her into bed with us so I could control what I couldn't control. What I could never control: my dignity in the face of someone I adore. Losing it was the first thing I ever learned to fear; the cause of all my fear. My Waterloo in love.

I am four years old. I am a very thin and little girl. So thin and little that my mother actually takes me to the doctor to make sure I'm healthy. After examining me, he allays my mother's fears with one statement that quickly becomes family lore. "She is just 'tin' child!" he declares, in his thick German accent. He suggests I be given more exercise to stimulate my tiny appetite. So I am sent to my first ballet class.

After school one day, a short while later, I ask my mother for a banana. (I now don't remember particularly liking bananas—I liked fish sticks and macaroni with ketchup—but on this particular day I wanted a banana.) The request is refused on two counts. One: we don't eat between meals in this house. Two: you won't eat your dinner if you eat a banana now. But I am headstrong in my desire and beg so hard that I am finally handed a large, bright yellow banana. It is longer than my face. Victory.

I go to the landing at the top of our staircase and look out the little picture window with my banana in hand. I peel down the top an inch or two and take a couple of bites. And stop. That's all I want.

My father, having witnessed the battle with my mother in the kitchen, comes up the stairs and tells me I had better finish that banana since I had asked for it. I know my father means what he says. Ten minutes later, he passes me and the banana again on the landing. The few inches of peel are now drooping around the few inches I have eaten, but the rest remains unpeeled, untouched. Again I am warned that I had better eat that damn banana, waste is not allowed in this household: you ask for it, you eat it. Daddy is very serious.

But being such headstrong little girl, I just will not eat the rest of that banana. Now comes the lesson.

As my mother looks on apprehensively—angry eruptions are frequent in our house—my father comes up to the landing, grabs the banana, pulls off the peel, and squashes it all over my face, rubbing the excess into my hair. As I stand there, frozen, I hear my mother cry out from the bottom of the stairs, "Don't, don't, I'll have to wash her hair!"

I don't remember anything after that moment, not how I felt, or what happened next—my mother probably washed my hair. But the quest for my lost dignity has become a lifelong obsession, a relentless search for the face beneath the banana. It's a face I've never seen. I was, in effect, erased from my own existence. It was the birth of my shame. And my rage.

This unfinished crusade has somehow led me here, to an obsession with an act of voluntary, disciplinary action that restores me to a sanity lost so long ago I can't remember it. I still love to control my food intake. And I have grown into a "tin" woman. A woman who has learned to embrace her terror of humiliation by choosing and desiring what to many is the ultimate act of humiliation: anal penetration. The weapon has become an instrument of pleasure in my adult world, and I am hell-bent on taking those last few inches of cock down my throat and up my ass. To this day, however, I don't finish a single banana without pulverizing it first in the blender.

Sometimes I wonder if the appeal of being ass-fucked, contrary to appearances, is that you can indulge in the naughty sensation of shitting on a man. When you open your ass enough to be fucked without pain, the sensation achieved, and then enjoyed, is that your bowels are open and you could be shitting on the cock that has been so bold as to enter. As such, perhaps being sodomized could be viewed as my answer to the banana, the ultimate act of revenge.

Out of the world of my bedroom, however, I fear that I will always be a little girl with banana dripping off her face, unable to forget that at any moment I am under the threat of humiliation from someone I love. The more I love, the greater the threat. When I am deprived by A-Man's absence or the possibility of his loss, the threat of real humiliation, unchosen humiliation, lurks nearby like a predator awaiting its prey. The waiting is agony and the perceptions of humiliation multiply like a virus. They become so powerful that I experience them as real and endure the same annihilation of identity my father accomplished wielding a half-peeled piece of fruit.

#291

As we approach year three, we approach three hundred ass-fucks. I love symmetry.

After eight days without his cock in my ass, I'm ready to be certified. Insane from deprivation. We arrange a Power Hour and a Half. Unusually, I want to talk and I tell him of my pending insanity.

I suggest to him that I am fully aware that he is not my answer (though my ass is convinced that he is). He concurs enthusiastically.

"I am definitely not the answer," he says. "I'm the question."

I immediately envisioned his cock entering my little asshole, his question firmly planted in the center of my being. I had it backwards, of course. My ass is the answer—for both of us.

He strips, sits on the end of the bed, knees apart, and puts a pillow on the floor between his feet. I get on my knees, and as sucking begins, my heart is relieved. He takes my head between his hands, I put my own hands on either side of his hips, resting on the bed, and he slowly, smoothly guides my head, mouth rounded, open and wet, down the length of his cock. Very slowly, all the way

until the tip of his cock meets the back of my throat. I give him total control, and become head and mouth for cock alone. It is so
slow and his cock is so hard, the edge of cement. Beauty flowed
back into my being and all my insanity flowed out like bilgewater.

Then he fucked my ass, only my ass, and as his cock began entry he whispered, "If you ever forget, remember this, this is the
point of connection, always."

SAVING FACE

I was, however, now making other connections.

When I confronted the mousy brunette that day, I asked her if she loved A-Man. I hadn't planned on asking, but I guess I wanted to know. Well, no, I already knew. But I wanted, just as she had, confirmation. My sadism (to her) and my masochism (to myself) were—perhaps more than at any other point in my life—each struggling for dominance. Her big brown eyes filled with tears and she murmured, "I try not to." And in that moment, all my desperate attempts to separate myself from her dissolved.

Unlike her, I was too proud to admit to jealousy or let her see my grief, but they were both there, like hers. No longer different from me, she *was* me, and I suddenly recognized what I had been searching for all my life—the face beneath the banana, the face of a little girl crushed and humiliated by love. My tears were rolling down her cheeks. And it was horrid. For weeks afterwards, I was haunted by that reflection of myself that I had never seen before.

But then the most astonishing realization gradually entered my consciousness. The brunette was, just as I had been, incapacitated, unable to act on her own behalf; she was not capable—not yet, anyway—of leaving her own pain behind her. But I was no longer incapable. I could make the decision for both of us, I could take action, because now I had the strength to leave the triangle, as I never could before. It was a kind of miracle.

What a strange gift this woman gave me, the ability to accomplish what all my spiritual searching, ultimately, could not—the ability to break the chain of pain, right here, right now. Not only for me, but for my fragile four-year-old self. She did, after all, live with me still. It was time to dry her face and take her home.

AFTER

ACCOUNTING

4/3/3/3/3/3/3/1/2/0/0/0/0/0/2/0/0/0/0/3
/2/1/2/1/2/1/1/0/0/0/1/1/2/3/1/2/2/3/1/
1/0/0/0/0/0

The above is an accounting of anal penetrations per week for year
three. All the zeros represent one of us being out of town. Except
the last five.

Number 298 was our last. The walls I had so carefully con-
structed around our love had split wide open. The world was in, and
we were over. I sent A-Man away. It was Time.

Yes, it was that sudden. That unexpected. Totally unplanned.
Time to end the pain, time to end the beauty: they had become inseparable, a sadomasochistic adagio.

So the search for the end of my end ended as abruptly as it had
begun three years before. A symmetry of sorts. A single, swift, clean
cut. No negotiations, no begging, no manipulations, no blame.
After #298—it was again a Friday afternoon—it was over with
A-Man while it was still hot as a volcano and beautiful as art. Try

that for courage. Though for me, it wasn't courage at all, it was necessity. I never would have had the courage to send him away.

Curious how another woman was always the catalyst for him and me: the Pre-Raphaelite had joined us and, now, the mousy brunette separated us. I must have much unfinished business with women, with my mother. But this is the Daddy story, not the Mommy story—or so I thought.

I started counting the zeros week after week after week, as if they would add up to something other than zero. Zeros marking the empty space in me where the nearly unbearable pain of loss grew and grew. I festered.

And I died.

The core of me that he had touched died.

I felt that I would grieve for him all my life. And I do. I had been grieving for him since the first time he came in my ass; why stop now just because he was no longer there?

If heaven is a taste of eternity in a moment of real time, then hell is an eternity of loss in a moment of real time.

Completely bereft. We didn't even make it to three hundred.

RECLAMATION

After many months without A-Man, the love bubble in which I had lived for so long began to deflate. I couldn't keep living like this. I used to be such a happy little sodomite; now I was a miserable little sodomite with only memories to taunt me.

There were some things to tidy up. I put the few clothes of his I had inside several plastic bags and hid them away. I resisted smelling them one last time, and in doing so, I knew I would have the strength to do what was necessary to move on. The few notes and photos I had I hid in a drawer, along with the small plastic bag of his pubic hair, the hair from that first trim. Nothing was thrown away, all was carefully preserved. You throw things away when love has turned to hate. That wasn't what had happened to me.

And then there was the Box. Sitting on my dresser, overflowing with the evidence of all I was trying to overcome, get beyond. I realized that I needed a bigger box—and one with a lock. There it was, waiting for me in the antique store: square, with a hinged lid, a red satin lining, and a tiny padlock with a key. In gold leaf. Perfect. I made the transfer, took one last, long, searing look, closed the lid, and locked it. I put the tiny key away. The casket was sealed—with tears, K-Y, and a wink to its future finder.

This shrine of sacred relics was my monument—to the divinity of my masochism, to the great joy that once so frequently passed my way, to a state of consciousness I can no longer access, to a chemical connection that reached far beyond any logic or rationale, to the sacred insanity that so blessedly pervaded my being. Now, where to put it? Nearby . . . but out of reach. Like a smoker's last pack, close by . . . but out of sight. Available . . . but forbidden.

Climbing out of love with him, I felt like a pelican trying to extract itself from an oil spill: lurching, falling, getting up, trying again. But even if the bird breaks free, its feathers remain saturated, forever marked. I realized that until the pain of loving him no longer interested me, I wouldn't be able to move on. Why was the pain so very interesting? It felt as though the key to my soul was buried inside it. The unmatched enormity of the ache begged for attention.

Taking solace in other compulsions, I made lots of lists. Lists of pros and cons. Lists of what I lost in losing him and what I would have lost if I'd kept him. Lists of what I have gained, what I have accomplished, whom I've dated. They meant nothing in the end, those lists, but they gave me something to do while I cried. I realized that I had to change in order to not want him. Who I had become wanted only him. I had to become someone else, yet again.

This is how my former self died, how I killed her. But she did not go quietly into the night. No, she raged herself into extinction with one last blast of scorching pain. Pain to stop the pain. But perhaps masochism never heals, just changes form. Different objects, different manifestations. I feared I could not be happy without my pain. But I had to direct it outside myself now; inside I was soaked to the bone.

After a while I started fucking men again—one by one. No longer obedient, I started telling them how to do it—"like this," "like that"—and they obliged. Having been slave to the King, I was all Queen with them, spreading the word to my jesters, even as I closed my eyes and pretended they were him. Every now and then it worked. And when it worked, it was worst of all: the tears streamed down my cheeks while they thought I was in ecstasy. Is not every affair after the Great One just another state of mourning, prolonged and disguised as some form of continuity or bravery when there is neither?

But I didn't let anyone else—and a few tried—into my sacred backyard. Now a tunnel of despair, it had become hallowed ground, a battlefield, now quiet, but filled with ghosts. If those walls could talk . . . I figured no one else would ever get in there. How could they possibly earn the right? Who could ever be worthy? Who, in their right mind, would even dare?

BACKDOOR BUDDHA

The loss continued, intolerable and relentless, and the other men only made it worse. I needed help. Badly. Peace of mind was a distant intellectual concept; I was crying every day. I had finally suffered enough. Enough to finally say "enough." My dignity was shattered. In an effort to wrest myself out of my self-pity, I signed up for a two-week retreat with seventeen hundred Buddhists five thousand miles away in an obscure part of England. To leave where he was. It was like tearing off my own flesh to escape the hold he had on me. Free, I had no skin. Like a burn victim.

The Buddhists I met were truly lovely people, welcoming me into their world without judgment despite the fact that I was probably only there for a quick fix in my moment of desperation. But even the wisdom of a quick fix, if it's Buddhist, can linger long after one's ego has regained its footing. And so while they all meditated on peace for all, I meditated on peace for me, feeling like the child among them.

Everyone I met at the retreat, all strangers, asked me with genuine interest how I was. And so I told them. One after the other smiled broadly at my tale of lost love. "Ah! But you are so fortunate!" said one man, beaming. "So very fortunate!" He almost looked envious. The explanation: any experience of great pain is releasing negative karma, and this release is nothing more than a cleansing, a clearing of the way to nirvana.

Well, while nirvana without A-Man in my ass seemed a most unlikely prospect, I had now become the one thing I wasn't before: willing. Willing to entertain the possibility of sanity without him, just as I had been willing three years earlier to entertain the possibility of giving myself to him for just one afternoon—and look where that had led me. One by one, over and over, again and again, my new Buddhist friends rejoiced at my great sadness . . . until the tears finally stopped. They just ran right out.

There was a young Englishman, also attending the retreat, who was staying at my B&B in the nearby town. Every morning at breakfast, he would smile at me as we ate poached eggs on toast at opposite ends of the communal table. Eventually we talked. He had been a devout Buddhist for eight years already, although he was only twenty-four years old. He even lived at a Buddhist center in northern England, where he was finishing his university education. Tall, with clear white skin, full red lips, and long curly black hair, he was handsome as hell; he reminded me of John the Baptist, whom Salome so loved. He was also kinder than kind, paler than pale, and sweeter than honey. And, I assumed, monklike—given his Buddhist devotion. After all, the one thing I thought would never happen at a Buddhist retreat was hedonistic sex. But, oh no, those naughty, wonderful Buddhists, sex is A-okay with them—so long as no one is getting hurt, and all karmas are properly aligned. Clearly more experienced in this than me, he began our alignment.

When I told him that I was leaving the next day, he suggested meeting up, after the evening meditation. I can't remember exactly how the proposition was phrased—it wasn't dinner or a movie or even a date—but he ended up in my cozy room with the Laura Ashley curtains, two narrow single beds, tea bags, and an electric water heater. Outside, needless to say, it was raining.

This beautiful Byronic Buddhist not only fucked me royally on the last evening of the retreat, but also performed a particular kind of surgery I had only vaguely considered being of any possible use. He became the second man to fuck my ass in my whole life— gently, wildly, eagerly, Buddhistically. It was amazing. The sex, yes, he was so able, so young, so ready . . . and then ready again. But more amazing was that it happened at all, that I allowed it when others had tried to no avail. But when he asked, I looked into his saintly sexy eyes and saw that he could be the one. The one kind enough.

It was like being vaccinated against the very illness I had so long been afflicted with. A-Man was the FirstMan, was the BestMan, but he was no longer the OnlyMan. The spell was broken. Buddha had found his way into my backyard. To think that God, that sly devil, had sent me a Buddhist John the Baptist to show me the way out of hell. Or at least to break the seal that bonded me to another but never to myself.

How does one let go of the best thing one has ever known in the hope of something better? With a crazy, illogical leap of faith. I left early the next morning, feeling blessed for the first time in a long time.

Time to shop.

HEELED

Upon returning home, I decided that I would not find a replacement or a continuation in a single man; I must find something entirely other. This plan got legs when I bought some new shoes. The right pair of shoes, at the right time, can really change a woman's attitude. And these weren't just any old shoes. These were the shoes in which I would find a new identity. Just as toe shoes had shaped the contours of my young life, these shoes would guide my life when submission to a man was no longer possible. These weren't nice, elegant, sleek Manolo Blahnik pumps. These were nasty, heavy, spiky heels—useful shoes, practical shoes. No more easy-to-lose mules for me; these were serious strap-ons with buckles galore. I like a shoe with a good metaphor to support me. Toe shoes, hooker shoes, it's all just bondage in the end.

I got a lot of shoe for fifty bucks. I called them my "Don't-Fuck-With-Me" shoes. They also, ironically, looked a lot like "Fuck-Me" shoes. Ah, the double-entendre shoes, the key to Freud's question "What do women want?"—"Fuck me!" but "Don't fuck with me!"

Black, heeled platforms. The front pedestal raised the ball of my foot off the ground two and half inches, and the heel, that gloriously slim yet strong heel, raised me up a solid seven inches. Finally, for the first time since being on pointe, I felt myself to be taller than the truth. But most important, my feet were far above the ground: it is the place where I am at my best in both mind and body. And, if necessary, these shoes could deliver a very healthy kick.

My new shoes became both shield and armor in the battle for a new way to live. I ended up buying pairs in all the other colors: silver, sky blue, and serious pink. Once strapped on, these shoes changed my entire demeanor. I became my own Amazon—Aphrodite, Artemis, and Athena rolled into one. A-Woman was born.

Equal in height to most men, I was now taller than many. I walked slowly, deliberately, proudly, stupendously on my shimmering, high-heeled weapons. Hope sprang alive as I peered about from my new perch. No longer looking up, I was looking down. No longer Slave, I was Mistress: the only refuge for a submissive with no Master. I started wearing my shoes around the house. With sweatpants, with underwear, without underwear, dusting a shelf, doing the dishes. One time I even shaved my pussy in the heels in order to do the dishes. Therapy. And I continued to rinse out my ass every time I bathed—a gesture of hope in a vacant lot.

Then, one day, as Leonard Cohen was singing "Dance Me to the End of Love" through the speakers, I started swaying to the music—"moving like they do in Babylon"—and I knew that I would be dancing again before too long in my "Don't-Fuck-With-Me" shoes. I was healed.

I had made the leap across the open chasm. It wasn't as wide as I'd thought. All those abbreviated M-words were never bridge enough to the other side. I never really liked being a "Miss." Too prissy. It was slightly better in French—"Mlle."—but still felt wanting—too petite for my budding enormity. Then came the opportunity for "Mrs." which felt horrendous, like my mother, and its dry, neutered alternative, "Ms." The problem with them all is that what followed was always a man's name—a father's or a husband's. Now I only recognize titles befitting a woman who belongs to herself.

Having traveled the long and twisted road from Masochist to Mistress . . . What next? Madam? Muse? And with whom? Perhaps with a man who is difficult to love. A-Man provided no challenge in this regard. Loving him was so easy, too easy; not loving him was hell. So perhaps the opposite: loving that is difficult, leaving that is easy. Would I not then learn some tolerance?

A-Man is now long gone. But was he ever really here? Did he ever really inhabit my ass and me? Was he indeed the demon-lover who avenged my anger, the ever-ready erection to which I so willingly and joyously martyred myself? Or was he the God of my own creation, the God I always wanted but couldn't have, couldn't find? Perhaps I finally found a place for Him, and A-Man entered my expectant space.

I believe the equation goes like this: sex can only be truly deep, truly life changing, truly transcendent if you are being fucked by

God; if you love your man like he was God. But—and here's the rub that no lube can assuage—if your man is God and shifts your world, then you are, by definition, in the very center of your female masochism, open, willing, vulnerable. A-Man was my God, but he was my Last God. I fear no man can be God again for me. Lucky for all of us, perhaps: less far to fall. But I mourn this with all my being; it is the loss, finally, of my insistent innocence. It has been a long process, the extrication of him and the excavation of my soul. He no longer lives in my ass. I live there now. What a place.

I have been to the precipice. I looked over, and fell off the ledge. But now I am back, back from the great valley of my masochism, back to bear witness—for myself but also for you—to my survival, to my return from a world where depth was all that mattered. If you don't fuck with death chasing you, you are mistaken. So long as love, crazy, crazy love, can be survived, there is no excuse. No excuse at all.

Go. Come.

Slowly, resentfully, I have moved out of slavery, though I cannot forget its freedom. But I am no longer blinded by obsession. I can now recognize what is commonly termed reality, wretched reality. I even live in it on occasion, when feeling perverse. I have endured the loss. Choice is mine. But I know what to do—and where to go—should I need a fix of beauty, of submission, of relief, of bliss. And, besides, I still have the Box. It does not only contain his DNA. It contains my very own madness—safely captured under its gilded lid.

But I don't need to open it. I have the key.

Acknowledgments

I would like to extend my deep appreciation to Alix Freedman for true friendship and to John Tottenham for being the first to say, yes, you must. I am eternally grateful to David Hirshey whose inexhaustible good humor and unwavering enthusiasm kept me laughing and gave me faith when mine faltered. And to Alice Truax, thank you for everything: guidance, intelligence, impeccable taste, and relentless pursuit.

I am very grateful to my persistent and brave agents Glen Hartley and Lynn Chu, and to Catharine Sprinkel for the handling of so many things. And to Michael Wolf, a lawyer with real integrity, many thanks.

At ReganBooks I want to thank—and applaud—Judith Regan, for her courage, Cassie Jones, who made it all happen on time, and Kurt Andrews, Paul Crichton, Michelle Ishay, Adrienne Makowski, and Kris Tobiassen.

And my great gratitude to all my beloved and delightful advisers and friends who offered wonderful suggestions as well as numerous pictorial responses to my work: Elizabeth Alley, Christopher d'Amboise, Jeff d'Avanzo, Erin Baiano, Beverly Berg, Jim Bressman, John B. Birchell Hughes, Laura Blum, Mary Bresovitch, Steve Brown, Leonard Cohen, Bonnie Dunn and Le Scandal, Alfredo Franco, Janet Goff, Bruce Grayson, Gregory Jarrett, Paul Kolnik, Elizabeth Kramer, Marc Kristal, Maureen Lasher, Gillian Marloth, Michele Mattei, David Mellon, Carolyn Mishner, Adam Peck, Quentin Phillips, Ray Sawhill, Michael Schrage, Michael Sigman, Michael Solomon, David Stenn, Neal Tabachnick, Bill Tonelli, Vicky Wilson, Leslie Zemeckis, Robin Ziemer, and, of course, A-Man, always.